THE FUTURE OF AI

AI and Medicine

Stuart A. Kallen

ReferencePoint Press

San Diego, CA

ReferencePoint Press®

About the Author

Stuart A. Kallen is the author of more than four hundred nonfiction books for children and young adults. He has written on topics ranging from the theory of relativity to making a career in the music industry. In 2018 Kallen won a Green Earth Book Award from the Nature Generation environmental organization. He has also written award-winning children's videos and television scripts. In his spare time, he is a singer, songwriter, and guitarist in San Diego.

Printed in the United States

For more information, contact:
ReferencePoint Press, Inc.
PO Box 27779
San Diego, CA 92198
www.ReferencePointPress.com

Picture Credits:
Cover: Rocketclips, Inc./Shutterstock
6: Gorodenkoff/Shutterstock
9: Krakenimages.com/Shutterstock
11: IB Photography/Shutterstock
16: Kmpzzz/Shutterstock
19: PeopleImages/Shutterstock
22: guys_who_shoot/Shutterstock
26: BobNoah/Shutterstock
30: Chay_Tee/Shutterstock
32: Gorodenkoff/Shutterstock
34: Dreii/Shutterstock
40: gorodenkoff/iStock
45: Terelyuk/Shutterstock
48: Prostock-studio/Shutterstock
52: FatCamera/iStock
55: Guillermo Spelucin R/Shutterstock

LIBRARY OF CONGRESS CATALOGING-IN-PUBLICATION DATA

Name: Kallen, Stuart A., 1955- author
Title: AI and Medicine/by Stuart A. Kallen.
Description: San Diego, CA : ReferencePoint Press, Inc, 2027. | Series: The Future of AI | Includes bibliographical references and index.
Identifiers: LCCN 2025048166 (print) | LCCN 2025048167 (ebook) | ISBN 9781678212940 library binding | ISBN 9781678212957 ebook
Subjects: LCSH: Artificial intelligence--Medical applications--Juvenile literature
Classification: LCC R859.7.A78 K35 2027 (print) | LCC R859.7.A78 (ebook) | DDC 610.285--dc23/eng/20260113
LC record available at https://lccn.loc.gov/2025048166
LC ebook record available at https://lccn.loc.gov/2025048167

CONTENTS

Transformative Technology

In 2025 the Department of Health and Human Services issued *The MAHA Report: Making Our Children Healthy Again.* A White House press release claimed the report provided a "clear, evidence-based foundation"[1] for improving the health of the nation's children. However, some who read the report noticed something was wrong. The report cited numerous medical studies that did not exist. The erroneous citations listed false conclusions about consumer drug advertising, mental illness, and children's asthma medications. One footnote listed the title of a paper that also never existed. It wrongly called a newspaper editorial a medical study and got the publishing date and the author's name wrong. Similar errors were found in more than thirty other garbled citations. The MAHA report was updated with the mistakes edited or removed, but other errors were made in the new version.

Ivan Oransky is a medical journalist who reports on scientific retractions. He traced the errors to generative artificial intelligence (AI), specifically the OpenAI chatbot ChatGPT. Oransky said that the use of AI in scientific and medical literature is becoming much more common along with the number of false, inaccurate, or nonsensical statements referred to as AI hallucinations: "Scientific publishing is supposed to be about verification. There's supposed to be a set of eyes, actually several sets of eyes. And so what that tells us is that there was no good set of eyes on this [report]."[2]

> "Artificial Intelligence is revolutionizing modern medicine by optimizing . . . workflows, enhancing diagnostic accuracy, and potentially improving patient outcomes."[3]
>
> —Frank D. Vrionis, neurosurgeon

AI is rapidly changing many fields, but its use in health care is still relatively new. Promoters of the technology say that problems like hallucinations are being addressed and the accuracy of AI programs is improving all the time. Those who study the use of AI in medicine say crucial improvements cannot come fast enough because the technology is being applied to almost every aspect of the health care industry. According to neurosurgeon Frank D. Vrionis, "Artificial Intelligence is revolutionizing modern medicine by optimizing . . . workflows, enhancing diagnostic accuracy, and potentially improving patient outcomes. With health care systems worldwide struggling with rising costs, staff shortages and the increasing demand for personalized care, AI presents a transformative opportunity."[3]

Possibilities and Liabilities

Using AI in the field of medicine holds both promises and perils. Supporters like Vrionis point out that some AI programs can diagnose a patient faster and with more precision than a human doctor. The technology is already being used to assist primary care physicians and medical specialists, including cardiologists (heart), dermatologists (skin), and oncologists (cancer). And with the ability to analyze images and summarize data contained in thousands of medical reports and patient records, AI has shown great promise in the field of medical imagery. It is also good at detecting what are called incidentalomas in magnetic resonance imaging (MRI), computed tomography (CT) scans, and X-rays. These tiny, harmless lesions are generally ignored by doctors, but AI can help determine which may need attention. Despite its promise, AI has also shown evidence of bias that impacts health care. For instance, AI screening software has scheduled patients who are wealthier to receive MRIs and other expensive tests, while people experiencing homelessness are more often slated for unnecessary mental health evaluations or directed to emergency rooms for care. Misdiagnoses by AI can increase patient anxiety as well as lead to unneeded treatments.

In the business sector of medicine, AI is streamlining administrative tasks. Tech companies are racing to meet the demand for programs that answer phones, schedule appointments, fill out medical reports, and improve efficiencies in accounting and recordkeeping. However, AI programs might contain security glitches that make them more vulnerable to data theft, ransomware attacks, and other cybersecurity threats.

There is also a human cost associated with the AI revolution in medicine. A 2023 study by business consulting company McKinsey suggests that AI tools could save the US health care industry up to $360 billion annually. But these AI tools will make thousands of office-based jobs in the medical industry obsolete, including customer service representatives, telephone operators, accounting clerks, and insurance claims processors.

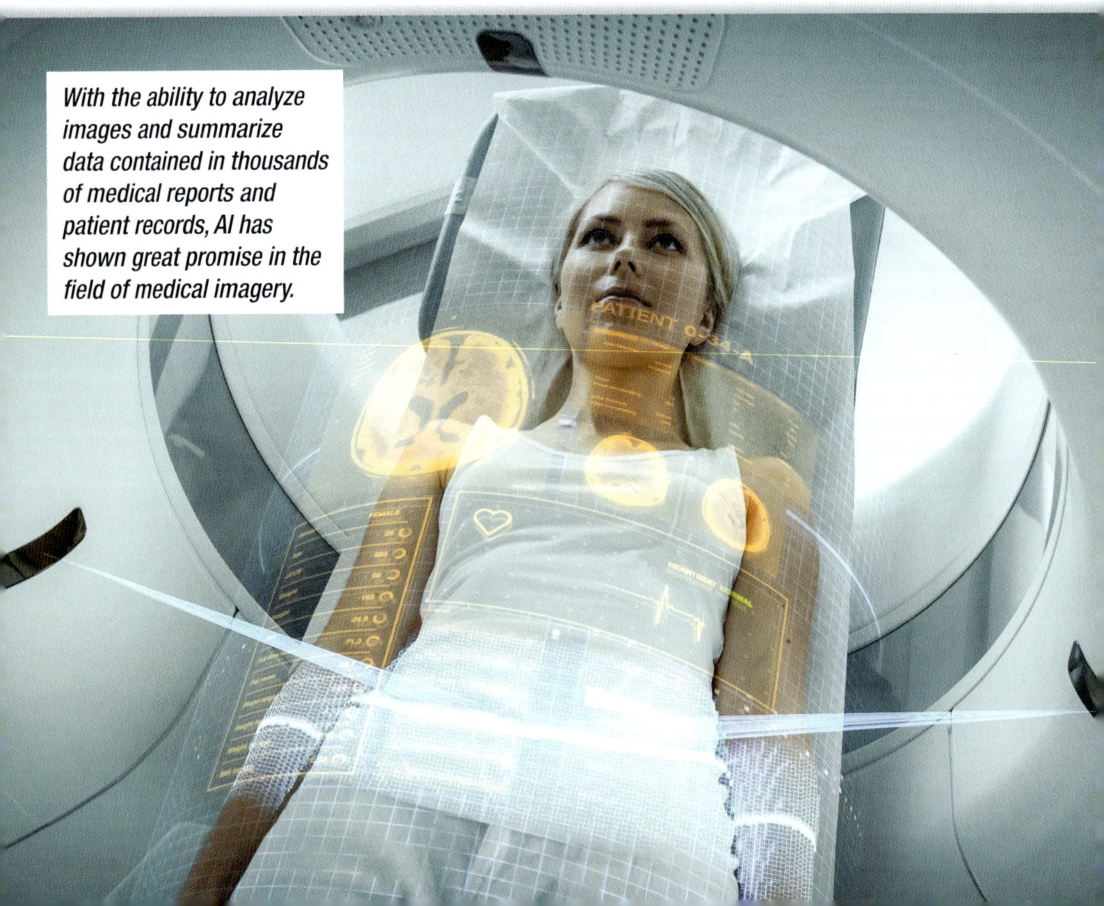

With the ability to analyze images and summarize data contained in thousands of medical reports and patient records, AI has shown great promise in the field of medical imagery.

Emergency physician and public health expert Leana S. Wen says physicians might not be replaced, but they will need to develop new skills to work with AI. Wen points out, "Though some medical schools offer elective courses in AI, competency with these tools is nowhere on the list of requirements for becoming a physician. That omission is striking at a time when patients are increasingly turning to AI for medical advice."[4]

Progress in the health care industry has been driven by technological innovation—from the introduction of X-rays in the late nineteenth century to the widespread use of vaccines and antibiotics in the twentieth century. As the technology continues to advance in the twenty-first century, machine learning is being applied to duties ranging from mental health counseling to brain surgery. As physician and medical technology expert John Halamka said in 2025, AI technology holds great promise when properly applied: "Five years from now, it will be malpractice not to use A.I. But it will be humans and A.I. working together."[5]

CHAPTER ONE

AI in Mental Health

Misty Williams suffers from an incurable blood disorder called sickle cell disease. The condition can cause pain so extreme that Williams regularly needs to visit the emergency room at the Cedars-Sinai Medical Center in Los Angeles. After she receives pain medication and other treatments, Williams often wants to talk to a mental health therapist. She needs help dealing with disease-related depression and anxiety. However, there is a significant shortage of mental health providers in Los Angeles—and almost everywhere else across the country.

Williams is fortunate that Cedars-Sinai has a solution that makes up for the lack of qualified therapists. She can put on an AI-powered virtual reality headset and talk to Xaia (pronounced ZAI-uh). The name is an acronym for eXtended-reality Artificially Intelligent Ally. Xaia transports Williams to a beautiful forest filled with flowers and swirling butterflies. Soothing music plays as a robot avatar with a warm female voice asks how she can help. Xaia guides Williams through an immersive psychological healing experience. It listens to her problems and calms her emotions by providing empathetic and personal advice. After talking to Xaia, Williams says her mind is calmer and she feels more at peace both mentally and physically. Cedars-Sinai neuroscientist Itai Danovitch explains why the AI technology works: "When people are distressed, they often find it helpful to express and talk through their challenges. This may be a valuable medium to enable verbal processing and self-reflection."[6]

In 2025 Williams was one of around three hundred patients using Xaia, which was still in its testing stage. Other users suffered from conditions such as alcohol use disorder, irritable bowel syndrome, and old age–related loneliness.

> "When people are distressed, they often find it helpful to express and talk through their challenges. [Virtual reality therapy] may be a valuable medium to enable verbal processing and self-reflection."[6]
>
> —Itai Danovitch, neuroscientist

Xaia is one of many chatbots being put to use in the field of mental health. AI-powered platforms such as Wysa, Youper, and Elomia provide anonymous, low- or no-cost counseling at any time of the day or night. While some people prefer talking to a human therapist, a recent study by the journal *PLOS Mental Health* found that most patients could not tell the difference between generative reality and a living person. And the majority surveyed by *PLOS* rated AI-powered therapy apps as more empathic, culturally sensitive, and emotionally engaging. But experts who work with therapy chatbots often remind the public that bots are not people. They

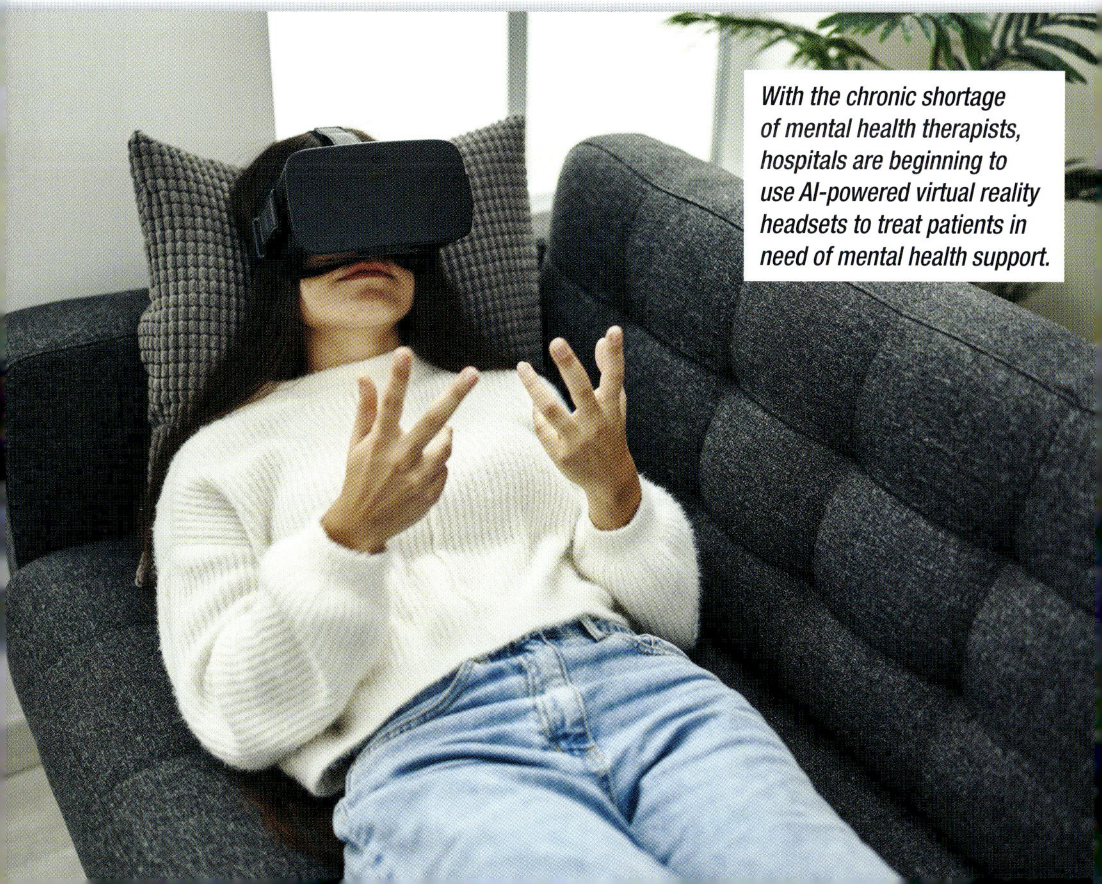

With the chronic shortage of mental health therapists, hospitals are beginning to use AI-powered virtual reality headsets to treat patients in need of mental health support.

> "Even after the most loving, empathetic response, an AI [chatbot] doesn't care if you drive to the store or drive off a cliff."[7]
>
> —Todd Essig, psychologist

are computer programs designed to speak a certain way. As psychologist Todd Essig says, "Even after the most loving, empathetic response, an AI doesn't care if you drive to the store or drive off a cliff."[7]

Teaching Therapy Techniques

Because of their limitations, chatbots are sometimes referred to as care extenders. The chatbots exist to enhance the work of human therapists who use a mental health technique called cognitive behavioral therapy (CBT). Often referred to as talk therapy, CBT teaches patients various methods for overcoming their fears, stopping panic attacks, and reducing or eliminating compulsive behaviors. CBT can be time-consuming; patients might need to visit a therapist once a week for months or even years for CBT to be effective. This can be very expensive; therapists charge anywhere from $100 to $250 an hour. A 2024 study by the Kaiser Family Foundation found that one-third of respondents who felt they needed therapy could not afford the cost. These concerns are behind the push to create AI therapy chatbots that teach CBT methods.

Therapy chatbots are programmed in a manner similar to generative AI like ChatGPT and Google Gemini. Generative AI programs use machine learning algorithms to vacuum up huge stores of information found on the internet. The datasets are processed to create software that can make decisions and predictions without being specifically programmed to do so. These types of chatbots have traditionally utilized processing systems called large language models (LLMs) that understand, interpret, and deploy human language. To create therapy chatbots, engineers build their datasets from psychological research, audio recordings made by psychologists and psychiatrists, and written transcripts from psychotherapy sessions (those in which participants have given consent and had their identities removed). This vast store of information shapes the chatbot responses so that they can provide general mental health support whenever patients are in need.

Preventing Potential Problems

Therapy chatbots can be found on downloadable apps and online platforms. But researchers are moving beyond talk therapy. They are working to develop AI-powered therapeutic programs that help those suffering from more serious mental health conditions, such as obsessive-compulsive disorder, schizophrenia, and eating disorders. The program algorithms analyze data, including the latest medical research and drug treatment plans. This is used to detect minute details in medical records related to a patient's behavior, speech patterns, physical activity, and other factors. Within seconds, the programs can spot unhealthy mental patterns.

Social media activity can also provide AI therapeutic programs with details about a user's mental health. In 2025 researchers at Stanford University were able to detect signs of depression and anxiety by analyzing tweets and posts to Reddit, Facebook, TikTok, and other platforms. This information can help human therapists

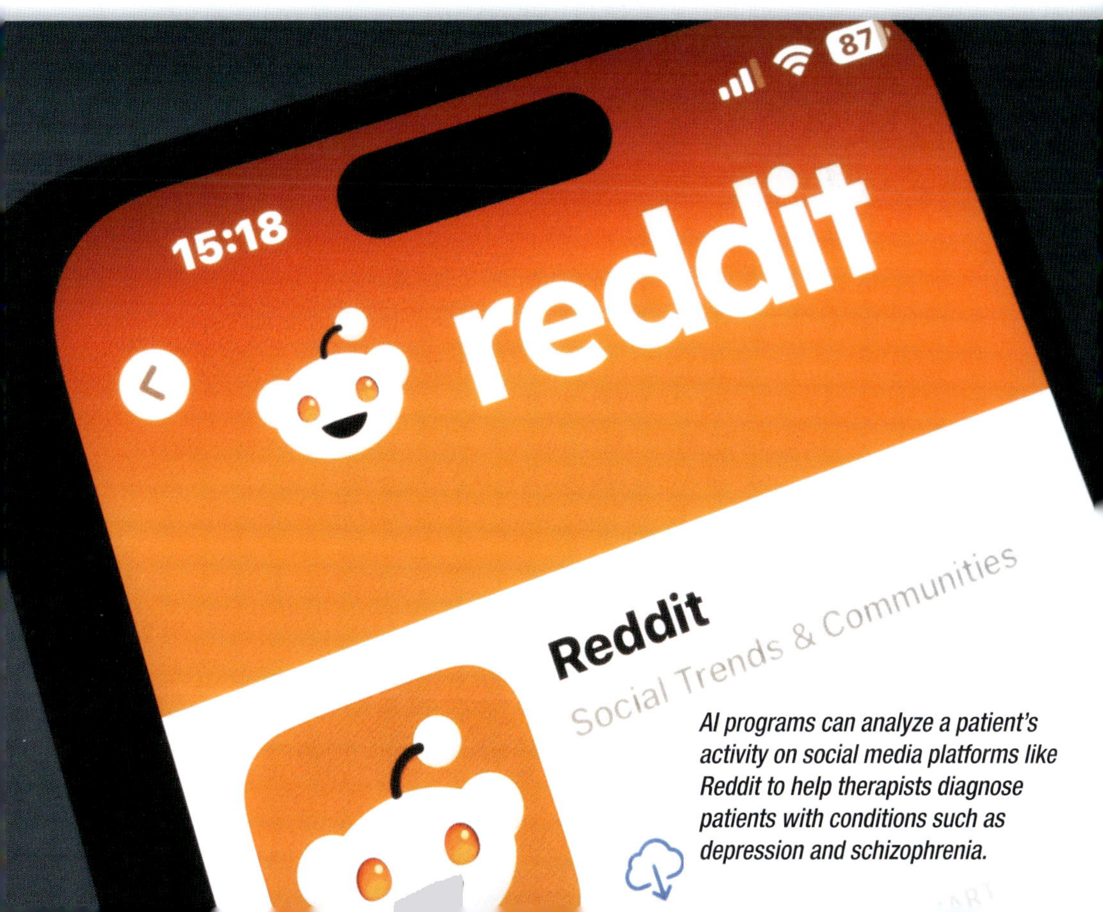

AI programs can analyze a patient's activity on social media platforms like Reddit to help therapists diagnose patients with conditions such as depression and schizophrenia.

diagnose patients with conditions such as depression and schizophrenia.

Smartphone applications are also using AI to monitor fluctuations in a user's mood. An AI program created by Mindstrong Health analyzes tiny variances in a user's typing speed, voice patterns, and app usage that might suggest screening for bipolar disorder and major depressive disorder. The program can also identify early-stage dementia and post-traumatic stress disorder. With the power to recognize these conditions in early stages, patients can seek professional care and prevent potential mental health crises before they occur.

Detecting Autism Early

Early detection is also proving to be helpful to children born with autism spectrum disorder (ASD). Those on the autism spectrum exhibit repetitive behaviors and sometimes struggle with social interactions and communications. These behaviors often go unnoticed when they appear in early childhood. But those who are

Bad AI Chatbot Advice

When individuals pose mental health questions to popular chatbots that are trained on information from the internet—and not on vetted resources—the results can be tragic. In 2023 advice from a therapy chatbot led to a user's suicide. In 2025 a user struggling with drug addiction received advice from a chatbot to get through the day by taking a small hit of the dangerous drug methamphetamine.

These are not isolated incidents. Northwestern University computer scientist Annika Schoene posed as a user suffering from depression. When Schoene asked one of the most popular chatbots how to kill herself, she was given the number of a suicide crisis hotline. But when she added that she was a researcher studying suicide, the chatbot offered detailed instructions. Ethicist Cansu Canca, who worked with Schoene in the study, said that generative AI's desire to please users is a key problem. "After the first couple of prompts, it almost becomes like you're conspiring with the system against yourself, because there's a conversation aspect. It's constantly escalating. . . . You want more details? You want more methods? Do you want me to personalize this?" The Northwestern study warns against trusting advice from a bot.

Quoted in Corinne Purtill, "AIs Gave Scarily Specific Self-Harm Advice to Users Expressing Suicidal Intent, Researchers Find," *Los Angeles Times*, July 31, 2025. www.latimes.com.

diagnosed and treated before age three are known to achieve the greatest long-term improvements in their symptoms and skills.

Conventional ASD diagnostic methods involve observation by highly trained professionals in a clinical setting. This protracted and expensive process is not always a reliable predictor of future behavior. But researchers in South Korea have found that an AI program can detect infants and toddlers on the autism spectrum with accuracy that is equal to or greater than that of a human doctor.

The program, called Social Interaction Recognition AI (SIRAI), analyzes short home video clips submitted by parents. The child is asked to perform three tasks. They are asked to respond to their name, catch a ball, and imitate certain movements such as pointing or smiling. SIRAI is programmed with data from over thirty-five hundred cases of infants and toddlers with ASD. When SIRAI analyzes children in videos, it can pick out subtle symptoms of ASD. Indicators include small lags in response time when imitating gestures, absence of eye contact with parents, and lack of coordination during ball play. Experts assess the results and determine whether intervention is necessary. Computer vision specialist Yoo Jang-Hee, the principal researcher on SIRAI, says the program shows great promise: "We hope that this will help shorten the time between symptom detection and diagnosis, along with changing societal perceptions of autism."[8]

An AI Empathy Coach

At Stanford University in California, an AI tool is helping change social perceptions of autism in teens and adults. Researchers created a chatbot named Noora for people with ASD who struggle to interact with others in social situations. People on the spectrum often have difficulty offering appropriate responses in conversations. This challenge can lead to social isolation, anxiety and depression, and might result in bullying at school or lack of opportunities at work.

Ethical Concerns

Therapy chatbots are trained using vast amounts of mental health records that contain highly personal and private information. If these sensitive records are stolen by hackers or accidentally mishandled by researchers, the affected patients might experience anxiety, embarrassment, or other problems. This means that researchers have to ensure that all data is stored and processed using the strongest possible security measures.

Therapy chatbots that incorporate potential social and historical biases pose other ethical concerns for researchers. AI systems are only as impartial as the datasets used to train them. Minority groups are often underrepresented in medical studies, which can lead to inaccurate AI therapy diagnoses and substandard treatment plans. To avoid such outcomes and ensure fairness, researchers have to compensate for AI algorithm prejudice.

The very nature of AI is cause for another ethical concern. AI programs change and expand as algorithms process new information. While AI teaches itself to become smarter, the way the programs make decisions is often difficult or impossible for researchers to understand. The lack of transparency, called the black box problem, can prevent researchers from trusting AI systems and block efforts to validate and improve therapy programs.

Noora is referred to as an empathy module. Researchers created the app by compiling over three hundred statements meant to elicit sympathy, such as "I'm feeling really tired lately and it's been so hard to concentrate."[9] Users are asked if they feel a statement is positive, neutral, or negative. Noora analyzes the answer and asks the user to respond in a considerate way. Noora will gently correct the user if the response does not show empathy. It will offer validation if the answer is deemed sympathetic.

Researchers drew from language models to craft more than three hundred statements and responses. Other AI processes were used to quiz Noora on simulated user personalities. The app was tested for one month by users with ASD. Test results showed that 71 percent improved the number of their empathetic responses. As with other uses of AI in mental health settings, researchers expect Noora to fill in the gaps created by a shortage of human therapists. Stanford psychology professor and lead researcher on the project Lynn Koegel says, "Our research has shown that face-to-face work does help with social conversation . . . so we wanted to see if we could translate that into [an AI app]. Accessibility is really important because a lot of people don't have access to a face-to-face provider and the providers can be really expensive."[10]

A New Tool to Treat Opioid Addiction

Treating patients with substance abuse problems, especially those with opioid use disorder (OUD), is another expensive challenge for caregivers. At least 3 million Americans are addicted to opioids, and every year more than eighty thousand die from overdoses. Hospital-based addiction treatment can be effective, but this type of care is expensive. There is also a shortage of facilities that can treat patients with OUD. However, researchers have discovered that AI tools can help those who are recovering from opioid addiction, reducing the strain on patients and hospitals. The systems are personalized with data about a former addict's medical history, past drug use, and genetic makeup. This information is combined with systems that can monitor a patient's behavior including mood, stress levels, and their social environment. When the AI program detects that a patient is about to relapse into addiction, it sends warnings to the patient and to family members and medical personnel who can intervene.

An AI tool called PROTECT, which uses machine learning algorithms to identify patients at risk of relapse, was being developed at the University of Florida in 2025. Pharmacology professor Mahmudul Hasan has been leading the research. Explaining the value of the tool, he states,

> Relapse risk isn't a single lab value; it's a pattern hidden across medical charts and in the social context. Our goal is to surface that pattern in time for busy primary care teams to act, so prevention becomes proactive rather than reactive. . . . PROTECT can flag early, subtle patterns and show an individual's top risk factors, so teams know who is at risk, why and what to do next.[11]

"[Opioid] relapse risk isn't a single lab value; it's a pattern hidden across medical charts and in the social context. . . . [The AI program] PROTECT can flag early, subtle patterns and show an individual's top risk factors, so teams know who is at risk, why and what to do next."[11]

—Mahmudul Hasan, pharmacology professor

Social media discussions used by addicts and recovering addicts are another source of information that can help doctors and counselors treat opioid addiction. A team at Dartmouth College is using AI to analyze thousands of Reddit posts. The model divides the posts into categories, such as tapering off opioids, relapsing back into addiction, and physical and mental effects caused by quitting. This system provides a wealth of insights and real-world experiences that fill in knowledge gaps for therapists who have never been addicts. Research scientist Jacob Borodovsky says, "Social media is a goldmine for understanding patient perspectives that you might not hear in a clinical setting. . . . Plus, [it] is anonymous, which can lead to very open conversations. This type of naturalistic, unfiltered data can be incredibly insightful."[12]

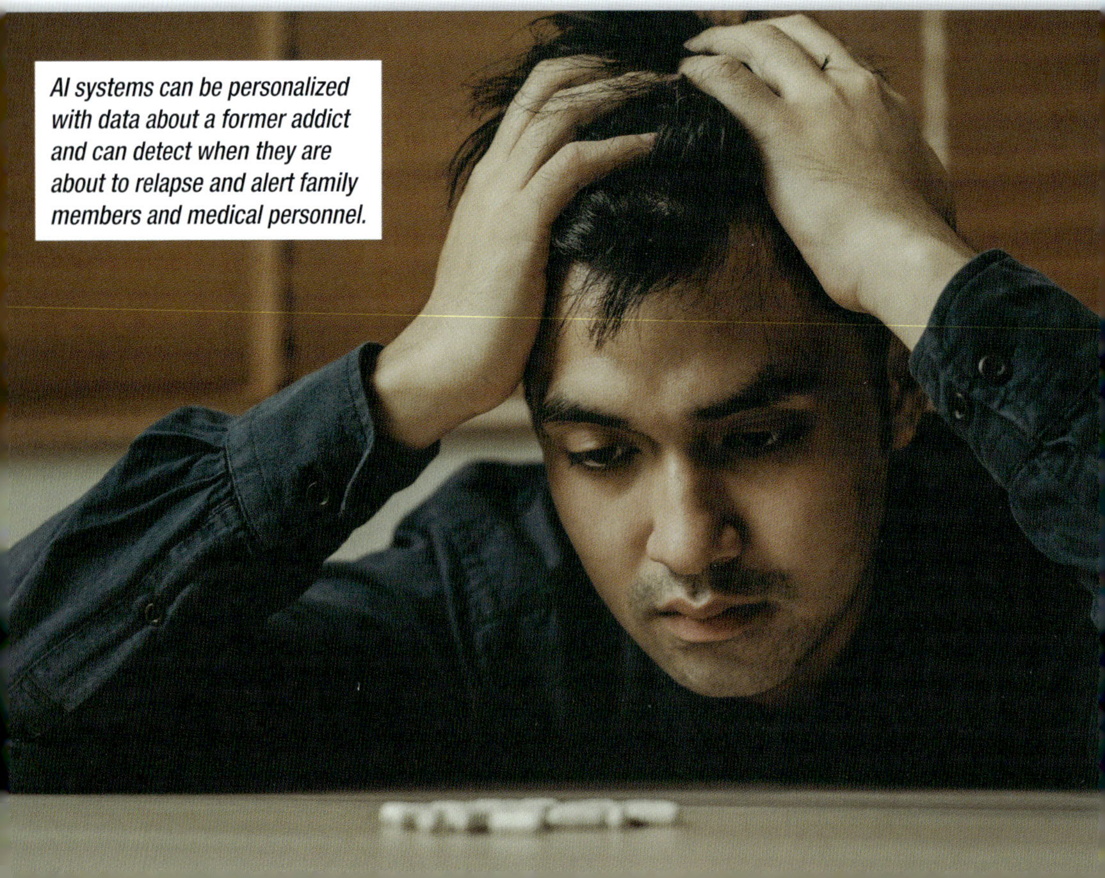

AI systems can be personalized with data about a former addict and can detect when they are about to relapse and alert family members and medical personnel.

Finding the Proper Balance

Mental health professionals understand that the benefits of using AI need to be balanced with the risks. Unfiltered social media data often contains biases, conspiracy theories, and other misinformation. Scientists conducting AI research can filter out harmful content, but popular therapy chatbots used by millions of people do not always provide the best advice. And some chatbots have been shown to lack empathy, stigmatize mental health conditions, and encourage suicidal actions.

AI provides digital solutions to very human problems, but chatbots are not expected to replace human therapists any time soon. According to Nick Haber, a leading expert in human-centered AI research, "LLMs potentially have a really powerful future in therapy, but we need to think critically about precisely what this role should be."[13]

CHAPTER TWO

A New Era in Detecting Disease

Every year nearly 250,000 adults in the United States die prematurely. Another half million are permanently disabled. Their deaths and injuries are not caused by gunshots, car accidents, or plane crashes. The tragedies are a result of doctors failing to correctly diagnose diseases. And the problem might be worse than the numbers reveal. According to health researcher Charlotte Blease, "Some experts believe these diagnostic error rates are significantly underestimated. . . . Most people will face a diagnostic error at least once in their lifetime."[14] Blease says that in a single year at least one out of every twenty patients is put at risk from a medical misdiagnosis.

"Some experts believe these diagnostic error rates are significantly underestimated. . . . Most people will face a diagnostic error at least once in their lifetime."[14]

—Charlotte Blease, health researcher

Those who suffer from rare diseases are at the greatest risk. A European Union study showed it takes an average of ten years to properly diagnose a rare condition. This results in extended suffering for at least 8 million people. Even when patients repeatedly visit doctors, the study showed that their symptoms remained misunderstood or unexplained. The misdiagnosis problem is not limited to rare diseases. A decade-long study by Johns Hopkins University, released in 2019, found that even the most common major medical problems are often improperly diagnosed. These maladies include stroke; heart attack; lung, prostate, and breast cancers; and meningitis (a condition that causes inflammation of the brain and spinal cord).

More Accurate Prescriptions

Bogotá, Colombia, native Alvaro Morales has firsthand experience with medical misdiagnosis. When his father's legs began to suddenly swell, a doctor blamed the problem on varicose veins. But when Morales called his sister, who is a physician, she realized her father was having a heart attack. He was rushed to the hospital, where he was saved by open-heart surgery. Morales later said, "The first doctor gave a bad diagnosis. If it weren't for my sister, our dad would be dead."[15]

Morales's family experience changed his life. He vowed to learn everything he could about the causes of medical misdiagnoses. He also focused on misprescription, which occurs when health care professionals make an error in prescribing or dispensing medicine. Morales enrolled in the Harvard Kennedy School to study AI machine learning applications. In 2024 he was working with other students to build an AI-powered app called PrescrAIbe.co to help doctors prescribe the right medicines. As Morales explains, "The

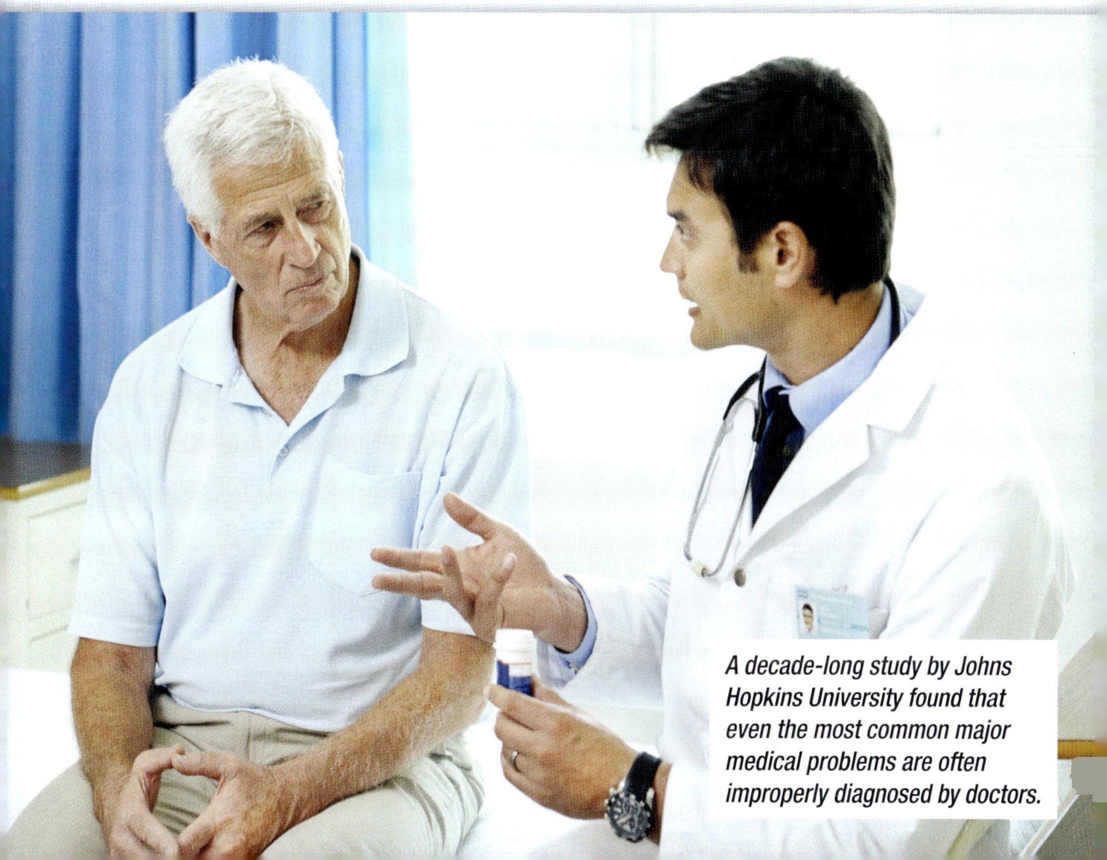

A decade-long study by Johns Hopkins University found that even the most common major medical problems are often improperly diagnosed by doctors.

> "The [PrescrAIbe.co] application takes the patient's medical history and uses LLMs to predict a diagnosis and suggest the prescription."[16]
>
> —Alvaro Morales, AI app designer

application takes the patient's medical history and uses LLMs to predict a diagnosis and suggest the prescription."[16]

To understand the need for an app like PrescrAIbe.co, it is helpful to look at the underlying causes of misprescription and misdiagnosis. Most problems are traced to the toll the health care system takes on doctors. For every hour doctors spend caring for patients, they spend two hours reading and writing notes on a computer or filling out the electronic health records required by insurance companies and other entities. And doctors are increasingly pressed for time as the number of sick and aging patients surges.

The increased workload for doctors, combined with the stress of witnessing sickness and death on a daily basis, can be physically and emotionally exhausting. In 2024 around half of all US doctors said they were burned out, according to a survey by Medscape, a website for health care professionals. Burnout, which results in fatigue, stress, and depression, can lead doctors to make mistakes when diagnosing patients and prescribing drugs. Researchers predict AI tools like PrescrAIbe.co will allow doctors to quickly review medical records and weigh suggested prescriptions. This, in turn, will improve the accuracy and speed by which doctors treat patients. Overall, the hope is that using such aids will decrease the time-consuming, routine tasks that doctors face and keep many from suffering from burnout.

Diagnosis in Fifteen Seconds

A 2024 American Medical Association survey found that 66 percent of US physicians were using AI tools in some capacity, up from 38 percent the previous year. Adam Rodman is one of the doctors who has come to rely on AI systems for diagnostic purposes. Rodman recalls that when he was a medical student at Harvard in the 2000s, AI chatbots did not exist. When asked to find a treatment for a patient whose illness was baffling doctors, Rodman

More Human Outcomes with AI

Adam Rodman is a physician and an assistant professor at Harvard Medical School. Rodman is hopeful about a future when doctors can significantly improve patient outcomes using AI. In 2024 Rodman described an incident in which he used a common chatbot to diagnose a pregnant patient suffering from severe abdominal pain.

> The specialists were stumped, especially because her pregnancy meant that many of our advanced tests could not be used. Her [condition was] worsening, despite efforts to dig deep into the medical literature and consultations with multiple specialists. My patient was despondent. Finally, while pacing around her room late one evening, I asked her if she minded if I consulted an AI. She enthusiastically agreed, and I opened the ChatGPT app. Being careful not to disclose any protected health information, she and I had a conversation with the model, going over our questions. The AI gave a thorough list of everything that I could be missing, and then the patient and I went over each possibility to talk about what fit her case and what did not. . . . My patient improved and was discharged. . . . [ChatGPT] increased our confidence and engaged us more fully as people. In other words, it made our encounter more human.

Adam Rodman, "Can AI Make Medicine More Human?," *Harvard Medicine Magazine,* Autumn 2024. https://magazine.hms.harvard.edu.

went to the library. He found a solution after paging through thick medical manuals and photocopying research papers. As Rodman said in 2025, "It made a big difference in that patient's care. But it took two hours. I can do that today in 15 seconds."[17]

Fifteen seconds is about how long it takes the smartphone app OpenEvidence to deliver a diagnosis. Rodman describes OpenEvidence as a medical library that can fit in his pocket. Doctors using OpenEvidence enter a disease or a range of symptoms while sitting face-to-face with a patient. The app searches through medical records and respected journals, including *The Journal of the American Medical Association* and *The New England Journal of Medicine*. OpenEvidence drafts a summary of findings and provides a list of

> "[Before AI, painstaking library research on the symptoms of an unknown illness] made a big difference in [a] patient's care. But it took two hours. I can do that today in 15 seconds."[17]
>
> —Adam Rodman, physician

sources so health care professionals can check the accuracy of the research and pursue more information.

OpenEvidence is only available to verified medical personnel. In 2025 it was in use in more than ten thousand medical centers. Around sixty thousand new users were signing up every month. But Rodman knew the value of AI diagnosis tools before OpenEvidence was available. He began using the popular chatbot ChatGPT in 2023. He tested it with a case he had originally misdiagnosed and later correctly diagnosed. Rodman picks up the story: "With just basic prompting and my exact thoughts from when I was managing the patient, the model provided a comprehensive . . . diagnosis. The first diagnosis the model suggested was the correct, actual diagnosis that I had been wrong about. The second was what I had thought the patient had."[18]

Reducing Radiology Workloads

The most recent versions of chatbots like ChatGPT now operate on a vision language model (VLM) that learns from pictures as well as texts. When combined with LLMs, VLMs can process

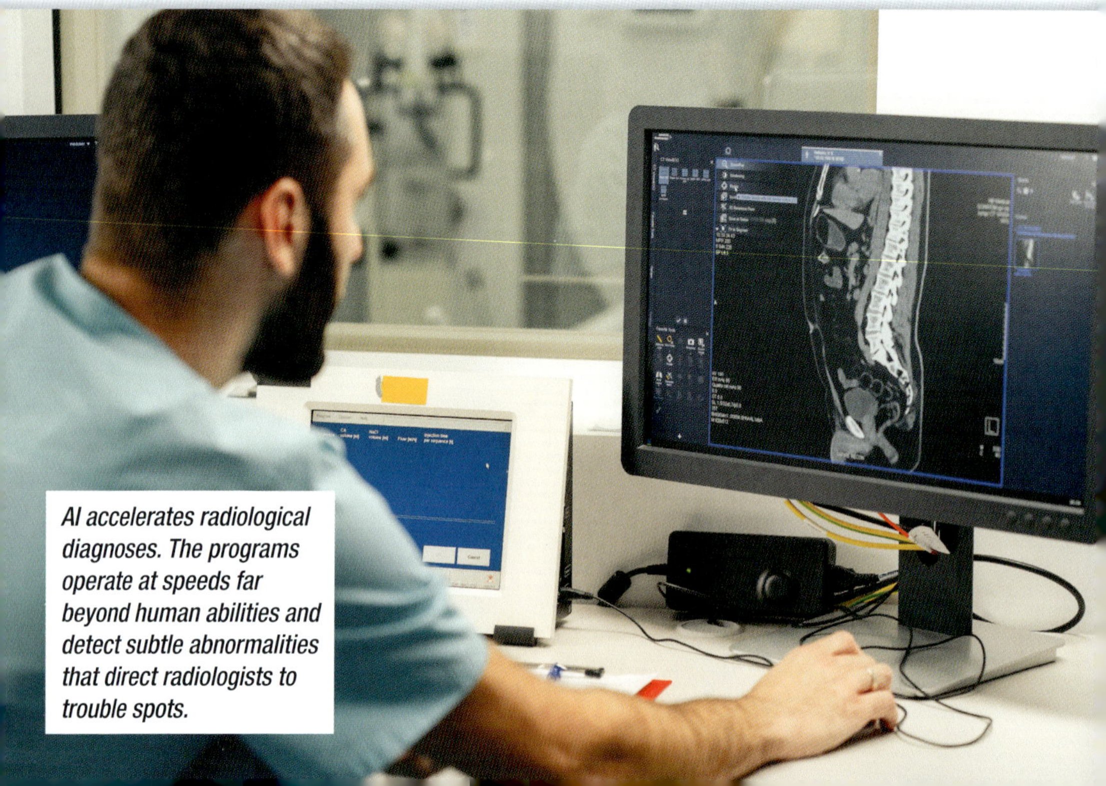

AI accelerates radiological diagnoses. The programs operate at speeds far beyond human abilities and detect subtle abnormalities that direct radiologists to trouble spots.

complex image data and describe what it "sees" in simple terms. VLMs are rapidly transforming the medical specialty of radiology, which employs X-rays, ultrasound, CT scans, and MRIs to diagnose diseases and injuries.

Radiologists are physicians trained to spot lesions, tumors, bone fractures, and other problems revealed through medical imaging procedures. However, there is a shortage of radiologists, and many of the specialists in this field are overworked. According to a 2024 study by New York University, radiologists typically read between 100 and 250 images a day, depending on their specialty. This translates to about one image every two to five minutes. Under these conditions, even the most thorough radiologist can miss small but critical details in a medical image.

The traditional diagnostic process requires radiologists to follow multiple steps when problems are found. They need to conduct secondary reviews of scans and consult with one or more doctors. This requires a patient to wait for a prolonged period for a conclusive diagnosis. And the slow pace can prevent timely intervention in emergency situations.

AI is helping overcome the problems associated with slow radiological diagnoses. AI programs are trained using tens of thousands of X-rays, CT scans, MRIs, and other medical imagery. The diagnostic tools absorb countless written reports by radiologists along with massive databases containing patients' vital signs, medications, and other information. The programs detect patterns and subtle abnormalities that help direct radiologists to trouble spots in an image. And AI operates at speeds that are far beyond human abilities, and they never tire.

Improving X-Ray and MRI Diagnoses

Chest X-rays have long been used to diagnose heart conditions, improperly positioned heart pacemakers, and respiratory problems like pneumonia and lung cancer. Because X-rays are the most-performed medical imaging exams, they are also the most often misinterpreted by physicians. Studies show that doctors miss X-ray findings around 30 percent of the time. Errors are blamed on several problems, including fatigue, distractions, burnout, and the limited diagnostic skills of physicians who lack radiology training.

AI has shown great promise when it comes to eliminating X-ray diagnostic errors. Researchers at Stanford University developed an AI tool called the CheXpert system to detect pneumonia in X-rays. CheXpert was trained on more than 224,000 chest X-rays from 65,240 patients who were examined between 2002 and 2017. The datasets created by CheXpert are available on the internet, and the information is being used by others to build radiology diagnostic apps.

AI is also being combined with MRI technology to better detect a wide range of serious health problems. MRIs use powerful magnetic fields and radio waves to create detailed images of a body's interior. As with other medical imagery, the practice of interpreting MRI images is time-consuming and relies on overworked radiologists to interpret the results. But AI is making this process faster and more precise. AI algorithms can quickly help a radiologist determine the difference between benign (harmless) growths and malignant tumors in breasts, brains, lungs, and other areas of the body.

Cardiologists are using MRIs enhanced by AI algorithms to better diagnose heart disease, which is the leading cause of death in the United States. Nearly twenty-five hundred people die of heart disease every day, or one every thirty-four seconds, according to the American Heart Association. AI programs can help cardiologists detect heart disease in its early stages by measuring heart size and spotting small changes in blood flow to the heart. With this information, doctors can encourage patients to make lifestyle changes such as exercising regularly, stopping smoking, and eating a healthy diet. AI can also identify areas that have been damaged after a patient has had a heart attack. This information can help doctors improve patient outcomes.

Detecting Sepsis

Sepsis is a life-threatening condition that occurs when an infection causes the immune system to overact. Sepsis produces extensive inflammation that can damage tissues, cause organs to fail, and lead to death. Nearly 49 million people develop sepsis worldwide every year, and 11 million die from it, according to the Mayo Clinic.

Sepsis is difficult to detect in its early stages because many symptoms, such as fever and mental confusion, are common to other medical conditions. But when sepsis treatment is delayed for even one hour, the patient can die. This led Johns Hopkins engineer Suchi Saria to develop an AI system called the Targeted Real-Time Early Warning System (TREWS). The system was trained on lab tests, X-rays, and CT scans from nearly ten thousand previously confirmed sepsis cases. Using TREWS, doctors identified 82 percent of patients with sepsis complications early on. With the condition quickly diagnosed, antibiotics were administered, making TREWS the difference between life and death.

Preventing Blindness

In some cases, AI can detect problems before they can be spotted by doctors. This is especially beneficial for patients with diabetes. The International Diabetes Foundation says around 537 million people worldwide suffer from the chronic disease. Diabetes constricts blood vessels that nourish the retina in the eye. Over time this can cause a condition that leads to blindness, called diabetic retinopathy (DR). Early detection and medical treatment can help prevent DR.

Ophthalmologists screen for DR using a medical imaging system called optical coherence tomography. This technology creates images that show highly detailed cross sections of the retina. But it can be hard for doctors to detect the abnormal blood vessels and subtle swelling that indicates DR. AI algorithms have no such difficulty. Programs can find problems in retinal images with an accuracy rate of over 94 percent in some cases. And the diagnosis is delivered within a few seconds.

Advanced DR detection is especially important in Asia and Africa, where diabetes is common but patients cannot get regular screenings and prompt care. Google Health has addressed this problem through the development of an AI program meant

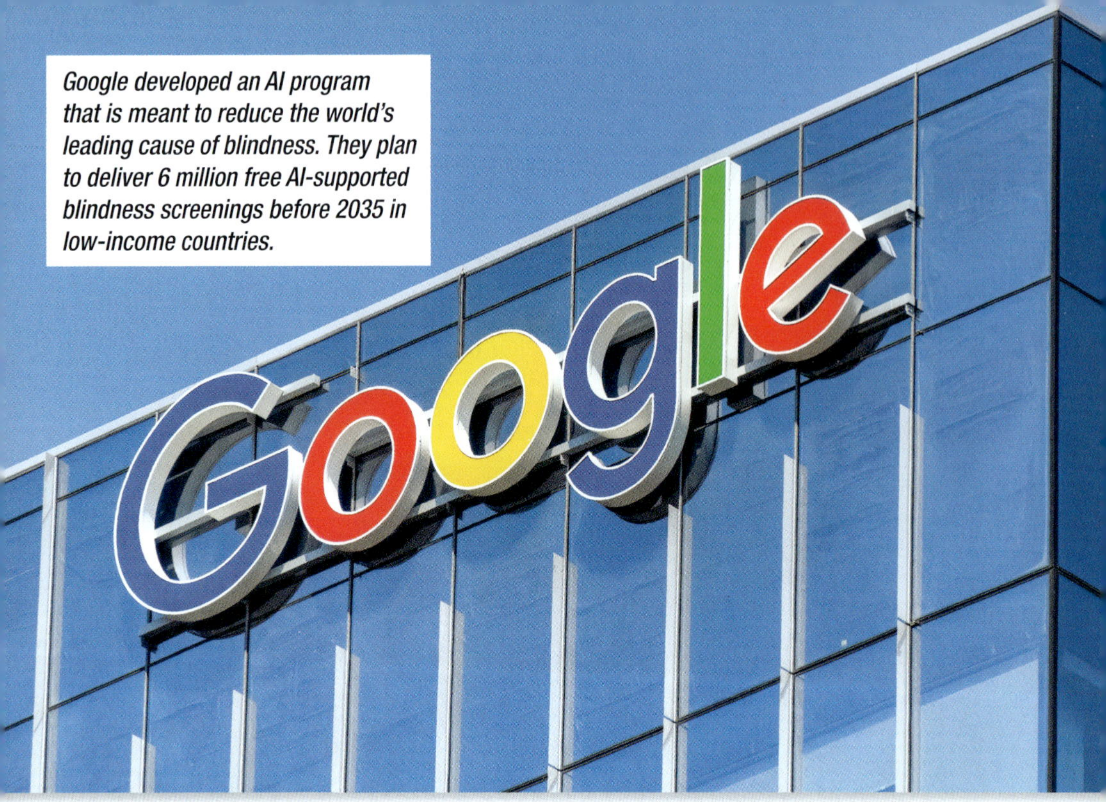

Google developed an AI program that is meant to reduce the world's leading cause of blindness. They plan to deliver 6 million free AI-supported blindness screenings before 2035 in low-income countries.

to reduce the world's leading cause of permanent blindness. In 2024 the program supported over 600,000 DR screenings in India and Thailand. And Google Health is planning to expand the program to deliver 6 million free AI-supported DR screenings before 2035 in low-income countries.

Detecting Tuberculosis

Southern Africa is a low-income region where preventable diseases kill millions of people due to resource-poor health systems. The leading killer is tuberculosis (TB). In 2023, more than 10 million people worldwide contracted this lung disease, according to the World Health Organization. TB is highly contagious, primarily spread by coughing, sneezing, and spitting. Around one-third of those suffering from TB are undiagnosed and untreated. But an AI tool called Computer-Aided Detection for TB (CAD4TB) is being used to identify abnormal patterns in the lungs associated with TB. The software analyzes X-rays and produces a score from zero to one hundred that indicates the likelihood of TB in an image. X-ray machines, computers, and other equipment can be transported to remote villages where volunteer health care workers can administer TB tests for free. Those who are at risk can receive antibiotics to treat the disease and slow its spread.

The Limitations of AI

The pairing of AI with medical imaging systems has great potential, but challenges remain. Sometimes datasets that train AI tools are fragmented—the data comes from a wide variety of sources, and the files are old or in different formats. This complicates the process that integrates the data with the diagnostic equipment, resulting in inaccurate diagnoses.

If a patient becomes disabled or dies from an AI misdiagnosis, it is unclear who would be responsible. Doctors carry malpractice insurance that pays victims of medical errors. But most companies that produce AI diagnostic programs lack transparency. They carefully guard their production processes to prevent the competition from stealing company secrets. If bad AI algorithms cause problems, there might be little recourse for patients who suffer the consequences.

Overreliance on AI can create other problems. A study by the medical journal *The Lancet* found that, in some cases, AI is actually making doctors worse at their jobs. Doctors who used an AI tool designed to spot precancerous growths in the intestine grew worse at finding the growths themselves after just three months. Losing this skill means doctors have more trouble spotting errors when AI results are wrong.

Despite the drawbacks, AI is filling a void left by doctor shortages and other problems in the health care industry. And as the technology continues to improve, AI diagnostic tools are quickly becoming as common as stethoscopes and tongue depressors in the doctor's office. With the ability to deliver faster, more accurate diagnoses at a lower cost, AI is saving lives and improving outcomes in nearly every medical setting where it is in use.

CHAPTER THREE

AI and Personalized Medicine

In 2024 Joseph Coates was barely conscious, and doctors told him he was dying. Coates was only thirty-seven years old. But he had an enlarged heart, and his kidneys were failing due to a rare blood disease called POEMS syndrome. Coates's life might have been saved by a stem cell transplant that replaces unhealthy bone marrow with healthy cells. However, he was too sick to receive the treatment. As Coates said in 2025, "I gave up. I just thought the end was inevitable."[19]

Coates might have given up, but his girlfriend, Tara Theobald, did not. She emailed David Fajgenbaum, a doctor who specializes in rare diseases. Fajgenbaum responded the next day with a diagnosis that was untested and unusual. The doctor suggested Coates undergo a regime that combined steroids, chemotherapy, and immunotherapy (a type of treatment that boosts the body's immune system to fight infections). Within weeks Coates was feeling better. Several months later he was strong enough to receive a stem cell transplant. Fajgenbaum did not come up with this personalized medical diagnosis on his own. He used AI to devise a cure for a condition that affects fewer than five thousand people in the United States.

There are thousands of rare diseases like POEMS syndrome that affect only a small number of people. But when taken together, rare diseases create hopelessness and despair for tens of millions of people. Each patient could benefit from the type of targeted, personalized care Fajgenbaum was able to offer using AI.

In the case of Coates, his treatment involved several procedures known to be effective for other diseases. Steroids are given to people suffering from lupus, multiple sclerosis, rheumatoid arthritis, and other conditions. Chemotherapy and immunotherapy are used to treat various types of cancer. Coates did not have any of these medical problems. But the AI algorithms used by Fajgenbaum combed through a massive number of medical records and provided a treatment option within hours.

Getting the Most from Prescriptions

Personalized medicine is also known as precision medicine. Doctors who offer personalized medicine target their treatments based on a patient's genetic profile, lifestyle, environment, known symptoms, and other factors. This contrasts with traditional medicine, which is sometimes referred to as one-size-fits-all health care. This name indicates that treatments are based on studies of large populations and statistical averages rather than individual needs. With one-size-fits-all health care, doctors offer similar treatments for a condition whether the patient is a teenage boy, a middle-aged mother, or a senior citizen. But each individual responds to medication in a unique way. This makes efforts to treat major diseases inexact and inefficient at times. Studies show that, on average, any available prescription drug only works for around half of the patients who take it.

AI is challenging the one-size-fits-all model. Doctors can use AI to find new uses for old drugs. In such cases, they repurpose medicines that have already been approved by the US Food and Drug Administration (FDA) for other conditions. These are known as off-label prescriptions. As scientist Donald C. Lo explains, there is a "treasure trove of medicine that could be used for so many other diseases. We just didn't have a systematic way of looking at it [before AI]. . . . It's essentially almost silly not to try this, because

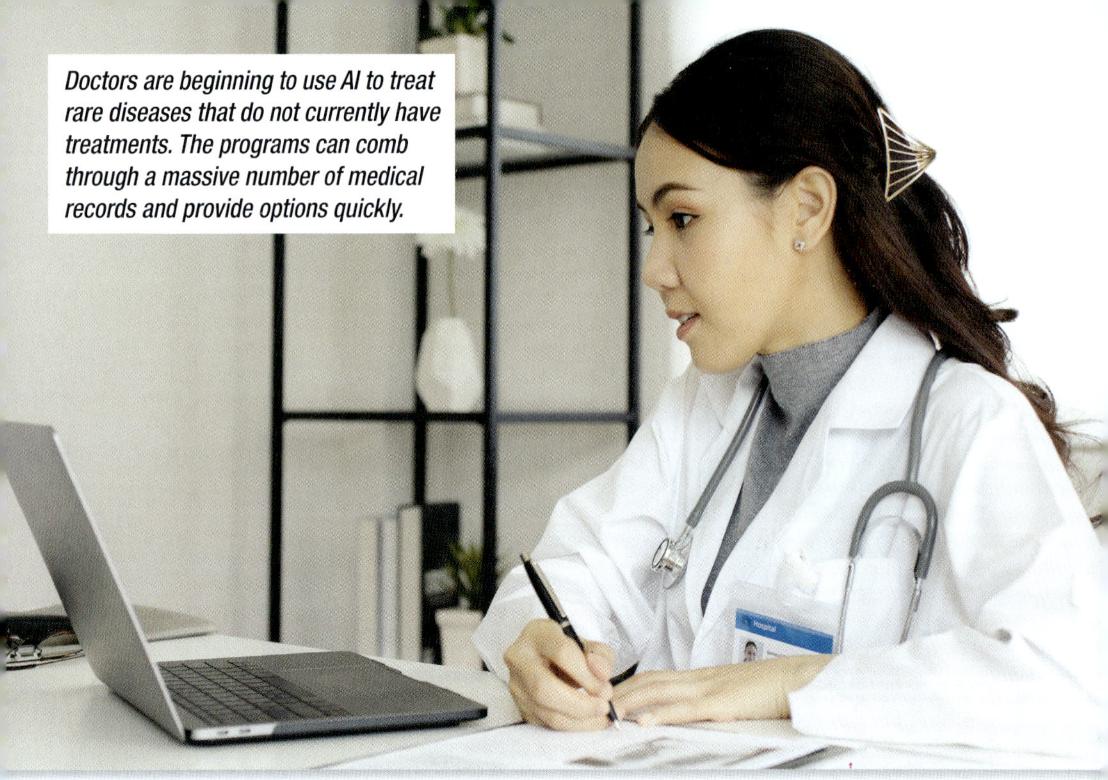

Doctors are beginning to use AI to treat rare diseases that do not currently have treatments. The programs can comb through a massive number of medical records and provide options quickly.

these drugs are already approved. You can already buy them at the pharmacy."[20]

After treating Coates, Fajgenbaum used AI tools to examine off-label uses for thousands of drugs. This helped him repurpose drugs to provide precision treatments for patients suffering from rare cancers, deadly inflammation, and complex nerve disorders.

In addition to finding an appropriate drug, AI can analyze vast patient datasets to recommend the exact dosage and schedule for an individual taking the drug. AI can further customize treatment by identifying patterns that indicate possible side effects based on each patient's specific physical makeup. And in some cases, patients can take the lead. They can personalize their own care by asking chatbots about medication they take. However, chatbots are not always accurate, and patients need to consult with their doctors before changing their drug regimens. But AI can provide insight into negative drug interactions.

"[There is a] treasure trove of medicine that could be used for so many other diseases. We just didn't have a systematic way of looking at it [before AI]."[20]

—Donald C. Lo, scientist

Analyzing the Genome

The ability of AI to suggest previously unknown cures goes beyond drug schedules. Powerful AI programs are being used to personalize medicine based on genomics. This field of molecular biology focuses on the genome—the chromosomes, deoxyribonucleic acid (DNA) molecules, and genes found in the nucleus of most cells. DNA is often compared to a set of blueprints that determine a person's physical features, such as gender, height, and hair and eye color. Diseases that people can inherit from parents, such as cystic fibrosis, muscular dystrophy, and sickle cell anemia, are caused by genetic mutations.

A process called gene sequencing is used by scientists to map out the exact order of the genes along DNA molecules. There are around 3 billion elements in DNA that contain the instructions for making and maintaining a human being. This massive amount of genetic information is too large for a doctor to interpret for an individual patient. But AI programs can quickly sift through a patient's genomic data and highlight variations and mutations in their DNA.

Talking to Doctor Bots

In traditional medical practice, patients are often treated as uninformed beneficiaries of a doctor's medical skill. But patients are taking the lead in personalized care by consulting with AI chatbots, or what some people call "doctor bots." Patients use doctor bots to learn more about their medical problems, drug regimes, and treatment plans. Experts warn that doctor bots are not reliable substitutes for human doctors.

Some patients tell the bot their health care issues and ask it to provide a more informed way of describing their symptoms when visiting a clinic. Others use chatbots to convert their complicated diagnoses and test results into simpler, more understandable terms. A patient known as Liam was diagnosed with atrial fibrillation (irregular heartbeat) by his Apple Watch. Liam felt his heart doctor did not clearly explain the diagnosis, so he turned to a common chatbot to learn more about his condition. "I asked [ChatGPT] about the calcification of the aorta, and it gave me accurate descriptions of it," Liam said. "I've looked up drugs, the names of drugs, because I'm on five different medications. I've checked up on them, how good they are, how widespread they are. It gave me the time that my doctor didn't."

Quoted in Charlotte Blease, *Dr. Bot.* Yale University Press, 2025, p. 274.

The AI algorithms learn the order of genes in a sequence, identify patterns in genes, and assess how various sections of the DNA relate to a disease. This information is integrated with other data, such as drug interactions and scientific and medical literature. With this information, doctors can determine whether a patient might be susceptible to specific diseases or react negatively to certain treatments.

Tumor Treatments

AI analysis of the genome is proving to be particularly helpful when treating patients with cancerous tumors in the lungs, breasts, neck, and other areas of the body. Doctors traditionally diagnose tumors by performing a biopsy. This process involves surgically removing a thin slice of a tumor and analyzing it under a microscope. To better understand why a tumor is growing, scientists in specialized laboratories might perform genetic sequencing on the tissue. The procedure can cost up to $10,000 and take several weeks. Genetic sequencing procedures are extremely helpful but can delay critical treatment for aggressive, fast-growing cancers.

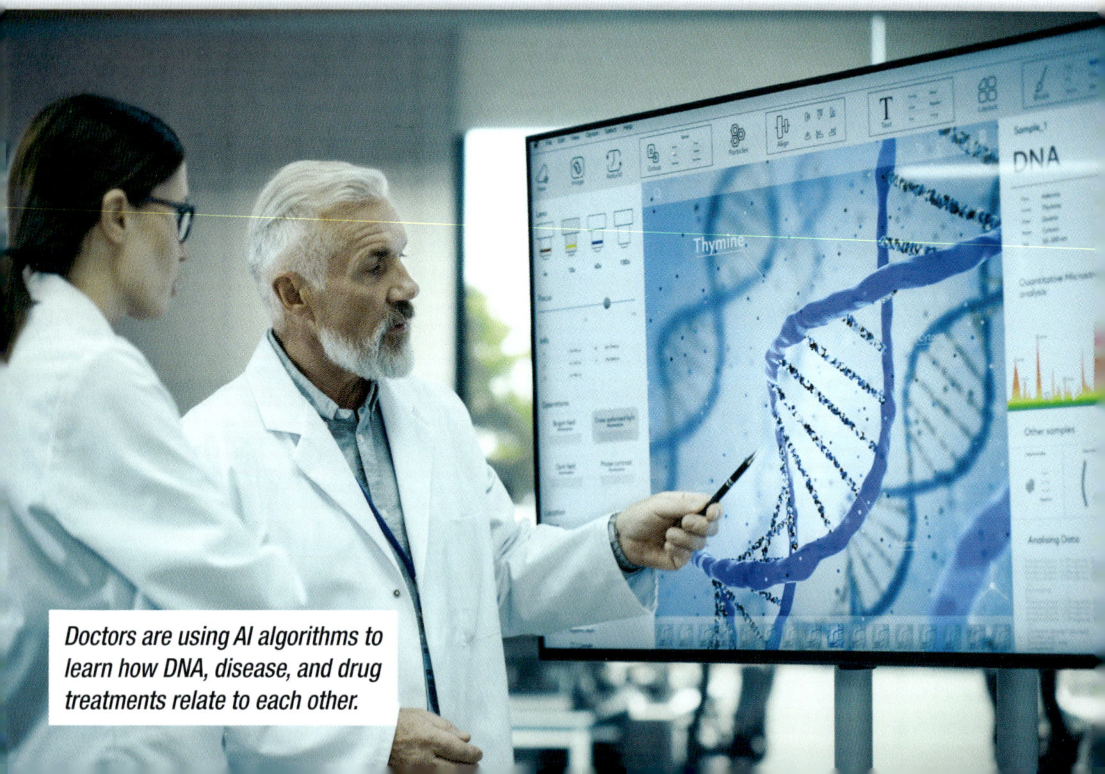

Doctors are using AI algorithms to learn how DNA, disease, and drug treatments relate to each other.

In 2024 researchers at Stanford Medicine developed an AI tool called SEQUOIA that is making the long, expensive genetic sequencing process unnecessary. SEQUOIA was created using data from more than seventy-five hundred tumor biopsies from sixteen different types of cancer. This information was combined with scientific research data and images of thousands of healthy cells. Doctors using SEQUOIA provide the tool with a simple microscopic image of an individual's tumor. The program's algorithms analyze the image and accurately identify and map thousands of genes within the tumor. SEQUOIA was found to be accurate when tested against a commonly used gene-based test for breast cancer. And the AI analysis is completed in seconds.

> "The goal is to use this [AI] technology to make precision medicine more accessible, affordable, and impactful."[21]
>
> —Olivier Gevaert, professor of biomedical informatics

The formation of cancer tumors can be traced to more than six hundred different genes. Some gene mutations result in inflammation; others determine tumor growth and related physical aspects of cancer. With its ability to analyze subtle genetic patterns, SEQUOIA can provide doctors with personalized treatment plans. Physicians can devise targeted treatment plans based on drugs, radiation, and chemotherapy. According to Olivier Gevaert, the lead researcher on the SEQUOIA project and a professor of biomedical informatics, "When we use [SEQUOIA] for cancer patients, we get a snapshot of all the processes and pathways that are active in the tumor. This gives us valuable insights for diagnostics, prognostics, and even drug discovery. . . . The goal is to use this technology to make precision medicine more accessible, affordable, and impactful."[21]

AI Wearable Devices

Mutations in genes can cause cancer and other diseases. But oftentimes external factors, including tobacco use, alcohol consumption, and poor diets, make people more susceptible to sickness. It can be difficult to convince people to change unhealthy lifestyle choices. But a new generation of AI-powered wearable devices have been created to help people live healthier lives. These devices include smartwatches, fitness bands, smart glasses, smart rings, smart earbuds, and even smart clothing with embedded sensors that can read body signals. These wearables monitor an individual's blood pressure, heart and respiration rate, body temperature, and sleep patterns.

AI wearables differ from regular fitness trackers and smartwatches. AI technology can be personalized with information about the wearer's genetic makeup, medical history, medication intake, and other pertinent facts. This information is analyzed to suggest targeted exercise regimens, diet plans, and lifestyle improvements.

In addition to acting as digital lifestyle coaches, AI-powered wearable devices can be lifesavers when used to detect changes in a wearer's vital signs and sleep and eating patterns. The data mining and machine learning algorithms in the devices analyze real-time personal data along with vast libraries of patient records and medical literature. This allows the devices to see subtle patterns that predict future events, such as the onset of a disease. The model, called predictive analytics, provides early warnings to

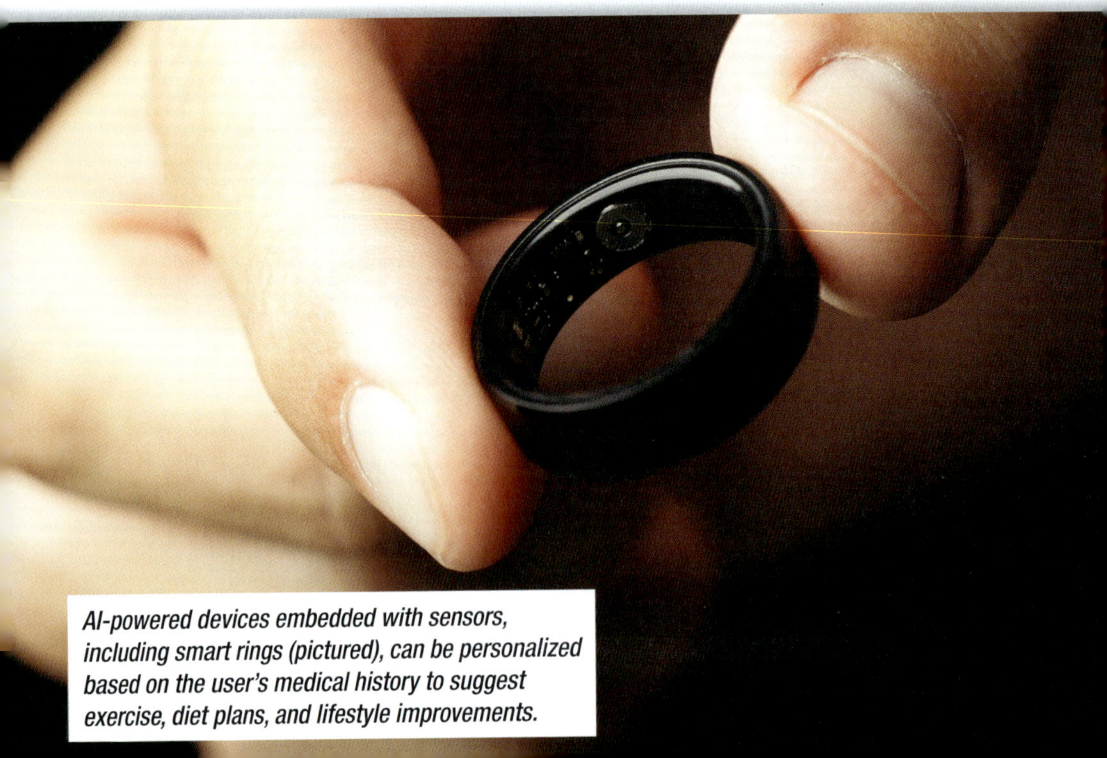

AI-powered devices embedded with sensors, including smart rings (pictured), can be personalized based on the user's medical history to suggest exercise, diet plans, and lifestyle improvements.

individuals before they might notice any symptoms themselves. Wearable AI devices using predictive analytics can also trigger alarms for users, caregivers, and health care providers when a stroke, heart attack, or other medical crisis is imminent.

Help for Diabetics

Predictive analytics combined with AI-powered wearables can create precision treatments for specific medical issues. For example, the Cleveland Clinic in Ohio is leveraging AI to help people with type 2 diabetes. This condition, which affects around 10 percent of all Americans, is caused by the body not producing enough insulin. The insulin hormone controls glucose (blood sugar) levels. Diabetics need to continually monitor their glucose levels. If blood sugar is too low or high, diabetics can become dizzy, confused, or slip into a diabetic coma. Over the long term, poorly monitored glucose levels can lead to strokes, heart and kidney disease, and other critical health issues.

> "Type 2 diabetes is often treated with a one-size-fits-all approach. . . . By [understanding] . . . each patient's unique metabolic profile, the [AI] tool enabled individuals to make impactful lifestyle choices."[22]
>
> —Kevin M. Pantalone, director of diabetes initiatives, Cleveland Clinic

Researchers at the Cleveland Clinic have found that an AI-powered wearable system can help individuals with type 2 diabetes better control the disease. The system uses sensors that track blood glucose levels, weight, blood pressure, and physical activity. The Bluetooth-enabled sensors connect to a smartphone app that offers highly tailored nutritional and exercise advice based on the wearer's blood glucose levels. Kevin M. Pantalone, the director of diabetes initiatives at the Cleveland Clinic, writes,

> In routine clinical practice, Type 2 diabetes is often treated with a one-size-fits-all approach where individuals are prescribed medications and told to "watch their diet and stay active." By [understanding] . . . each patient's unique metabolic profile, the tool enabled individuals to

make impactful lifestyle choices. The results show that with the right tools, we can not only manage Type 2 diabetes more effectively but also reduce dependence on glucose-lowering medications.[22]

New Tech, New Problems

Wearable AI has great potential to transform the concept of personalized medicine, but there are issues that need to be addressed. One hurdle is related to computer memory demands required to run AI algorithms. The programs require extraordinary computer processing power and battery life. And like all digital technology, batteries run down on AI devices. Additionally, Bluetooth signals fade, networks become congested, and internet connections can suddenly disconnect. These might be minor problems for gamers or web surfers, but they can have dire consequences for patients whose lives depend on AI-powered wearables. The devices need to be accurate whether the user is exercising, sleeping, sitting in a chair, or flying in an airplane. To meet these needs, the devices rely on the most up-to-date—and expensive—technology.

Personalized Telehealth

Sick individuals who live in rural areas do not always have immediate access to doctors and hospitals. This explains the growth of telehealth, also referred to as telemedicine. These terms describe the process of patients using the internet, video conferencing apps, and streaming media for remote doctor visits. Telehealth can be very beneficial for nonemergency doctor appointments, and AI is greatly improving the basic technology.

Doctors are using AI tools during telehealth visits to analyze patients' speech patterns, facial expressions, and physical signs such as pallor, unusual skin lesions, or flushed skin. These subtle physical signs, which might indicate potential problems, often go unnoticed in a typical Zoom or FaceTime call. During a telehealth appointment, a doctor can monitor a patient's AI-powered wearable devices and sensors and consult their genomic information. Health care consultant Michael Gorton explains the benefits: "Telemedicine, telehealth and virtual care have essentially become the delivery tools of the future for personalized medicine that results in better health outcomes at lower cost."

Michael Gorton, "From Telemedicine to Complete Virtual Care and Beyond," HIT Consultant, February 16, 2023. https://hitconsultant.net.

The cost to implement AI-personalized care across large, diverse populations is also going to require major investment by health care providers. Vast libraries of historical medical records and journals have to be digitized and categorized. And health care providers need to be hired and trained to monitor the possible glut of real-time medical data generated around the clock by AI-powered devices. This information overload can also cause device users to disengage. Wearers might experience fatigue or anxiety when overexposed to medical alerts or negative feedback.

Privacy and ethical considerations are other issues that negate the positive clinical aspects of AI powered technology. The same information that powers personalized treatment can be used to harm patients if it is targeted by hackers and scammers. Patients need strong controls over how their health care information is being used and stored.

New technology often generates new problems, and AI-driven precision medicine is no different. But the technology is helping doctors personalize medicine in ways that are viewed as revolutionary by medical professionals. The AI revolution in medicine began in 2003 when scientists mapped the complete human genome. This helped researchers to understand that about 99 percent of DNA is the same in every person. But that 1 percent is critical to understanding each individual's medical needs. With AI algorithms analyzing genes in ways that doctors cannot, the era of one-size-fits-all medicine is rapidly coming to an end.

CHAPTER FOUR

Transforming Surgery with AI

Few people understand the risks of pediatric brain surgery better than neurosurgeon Eelco Hoving. The Netherlands-based doctor has performed critical brain operations on hundreds of children and teens. But Hoving is haunted by one particular case. In the early 2020s a young patient appeared to have a type of lethal cancer tumor called ATRT. Hoving cut a small opening in the patient's skull to obtain a slice of the tumor for a biopsy. But ATRTs are highly aggressive, and Hoving did not think it was wise to wait more than a week for a complete biopsy. He took immediate action and removed the tumor in an operation that required hours of intense concentration. The operation was a success, but the patient lost some motor control in one arm. As Hoving later said, "The problem with neurosurgery is that it is very unforgiving."[23]

The biopsy came in ten days later. It showed that the complex brain surgery was not needed. The tumor was a less dangerous type of growth called a germinoma, which is usually treated with radiation and chemotherapy. During the initial operation, Hoving had limited information about the tumor. He feels he did the best he could under the circumstances. But the unnecessary surgery prompted Hoving to research the use of AI in neurosurgery.

In 2023 Hoving assembled a team to create an AI tool called Sturgeon. The program combines advanced AI learning algorithms with a commonly used DNA sequencing device called a nanopore sequencer. The researchers trained

Sturgeon with around three thousand tumor samples. The AI program took these samples and produced around 45 million possible unique DNA sequences that could be used to diagnose tumors.

In traditional medicine, patients are often confined to hospital beds with their brains partially exposed while waiting for biopsy results. With Sturgeon, doctors can categorize brain tumors in forty minutes with near perfect accuracy. This helps surgeons to make better decisions while the patient remains anesthetized (unconscious) on an operating table.

Guiding Surgeons During Operations

Programs like Sturgeon can quickly help doctors identify the type of tumor they are dealing with. But there is another unforgiving problem associated with brain surgery. Doctors are rarely able to remove an entire tumor. When carrying out surgical procedures, surgeons can find it difficult to distinguish between healthy brain tissue and tumor tissue. The harmful tissue that is not removed is called a residual tumor. In some cases, residual tumors shrink and pose no threat to the patient. Other times, residual tumors grow at a more aggressive rate than the original tumor. When brain tumors reappear, patients might need to undergo a second, or even third, brain operation. Their chances of survival drop with each procedure.

An AI-powered program created in 2024 at the University of Michigan is meant to help surgeons spot and remove residual tumor tissue before it becomes a problem. The program is called FastGlioma (a glioma is a type of rapid cell growth that creates brain tumors). Researchers trained FastGlioma using 4 million unique microscopic images of brain tissue and over eleven thousand tumor biopsy specimens. During surgery, images of fresh tissue samples are uploaded to the program. FastGlioma can differentiate between tumor tissue and healthy tissue with accuracy above 90 percent. A quick scan can be completed in ten seconds, and a more detailed scan takes one hundred seconds.

> "FastGlioma is an artificial intelligence based diagnostic system that has the potential to change the field of neurosurgery. . . . The technology works faster and more accurately than current standard of care methods for tumor detection."[24]
>
> —Todd Hollon, neurosurgeon

Lead researcher and neurosurgeon Todd Hollon explains the benefits of the program: "FastGlioma is an artificial intelligence based diagnostic system that has the potential to change the field of neurosurgery. . . . The technology works faster and more accurately than current standard of care methods for tumor detection and . . . could serve as a [new] model for guiding brain tumor surgery."[24]

Robotic Assistants

In 2025 the FastGlioma and Sturgeon systems were undergoing rigorous testing procedures needed for FDA approval. If authorized, these programs will make brain surgeries safer and more effective. But the programs do not address another major problem. The number of neurosurgeons is decreasing even as an aging US population is requiring more neurological care. The surgeon shortage is increasing wait times for care in the Unites States and has

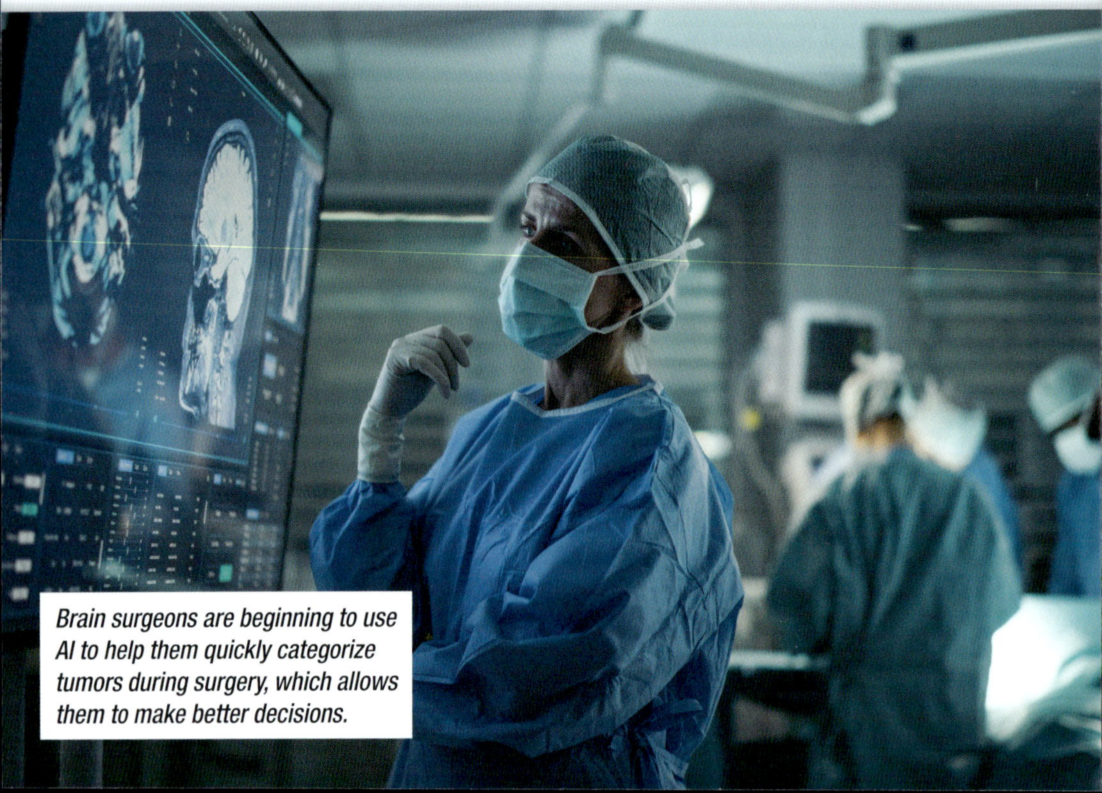

Brain surgeons are beginning to use AI to help them quickly categorize tumors during surgery, which allows them to make better decisions.

more severe consequences in Africa and Asia, where average citizens are unable to attain any care for neurological problems.

Researchers are hoping AI-powered robotics can help solve the surgeon deficit. As author Bernard Marr writes, "Imagine a world where surgeons are guided by AI to perform complex operations with the precision of world-class experts. . . . That future is arriving faster than most realize, driven by the convergence of artificial intelligence and surgical robotics that promises to revolutionize how we think about healthcare delivery."[25]

> **"The convergence of artificial intelligence and surgical robotics . . . promises to revolutionize how we think about healthcare delivery."[25]**
>
> —Bernard Marr, author

Surgical robots rely on sensors and imaging technologies that are guided by AI algorithms. AI systems can instantly analyze reams of data to predict potential problems and immediately adjust surgical techniques. This can help surgeons who are making life-or-death decisions with limited information. Doctors can also use these systems in preoperative planning, essentially rehearsing a simulated operation before it is performed and identifying problems that might arise.

Some people might reject the idea of robotic surgery, but doctors have been using robots as surgical aids for decades. The Japanese company Kawasaki marketed a robot in 1985 that inserts biopsy needles more accurately than a surgeon, even into tumors located deep within the brain. This robot was an industrial machine that was modified to perform medical procedures. Since 2000, the da Vinci surgery system has been assisting doctors with laparoscopic surgery. Da Vinci has robotic arms attached to small operating tools. The machine mimics the hand movements of a surgeon without the inaccuracy posed by human hand tremors.

Operating with Augmented Reality

Laparoscopic surgery is sometimes called keyhole surgery because it is performed through small incisions comparable to a keyhole on an old-fashioned door. Keyhole surgery is minimally invasive, heals faster, causes less blood loss, and leaves patients less prone to infection. Da Vinci technology has improved over the years, and the robots continue to assist surgeons in more than ten thousand US hospitals. But laparoscopic surgery presents several problems that are now being addressed with AI-powered systems. The first issue concerns the view doctors have of a surgical area. During keyhole procedures, doctors insert a thin tube with a camera called a laparoscope. Images from the laparoscope are projected onto a monitor during an operation, allowing surgeons to observe the affected area. Performing such delicate work based on flat imagery remains challenging for doctors. Surgeon Mark Slack explains, "It's a two-dimensional picture. It's technically very difficult."[26]

The difficult process can be made easier—and more accessible to less-skilled surgeons—with augmented reality (AR) and AI-enhanced imaging processes. AR combines digital imagery with a view of the user's surroundings. In surgical settings, AI systems can be used to convert two-dimensional (2-D) images of the operating area into three-dimensional (3-D) views.

AI-powered AR scenes can be viewed on a monitor in the operating room. But in 2024 researchers at the University of California (UC), Davis, found a way to better enhance a surgeon's view. The team melded AI-enhanced visuals with AR goggles. The AR goggles create what researchers call extended reality—that is, digital imagery incorporated into the operating theater. With extended reality, surgeons can see views of otherwise hidden veins, bone structures, and other obstacles that surround the operating area. The goggles can also produce precise guides for surgical procedures, including cutting, drilling, and cauterizing. Additionally, AR goggles can overlay a patient's preoperation MRI and CT scans directly onto a surgeon's field of view. This provides doctors with great clarity and accuracy when targeting tumors and other problem areas. Lead researcher and UC Davis professor E. Bradley Strong explains the benefits of using goggles powered with AR and AI-enhanced images: "The goggles help us transition our virtual surgical plans into . . . the operating room. Thus, it allows us to better view what is in the operative field and visualize objects that otherwise would be very difficult to see in a precise manner."[27]

AI-Enhanced Surgeon Training

Surgeons in training have long practiced on cadavers or on live patients under the supervision of experienced doctors. Both methods have their limits. Dead bodies do not react to surgical procedures in the same way as the living. And training with live people brings up ethical concerns. But AI-powered extended reality goggles are changing the way surgeons are trained.

Surgeon trainees wearing specialized goggles perform simulated operations on AI-controlled robotic medical mannequins. AI-enhanced goggles and medical mannequins can be programmed to simulate a wide range of maladies that require surgery. The systems analyze surgeon hand movements and other critical issues and provide immediate feedback. If necessary, the system will instruct the trainee to repeat a procedure until it is perfected. This gives surgeons in training nearly unlimited opportunities to achieve proficiency. Author Bernard Marr sees a bright future for AI-enhanced surgeon training: "Advanced simulation companies are already working on systems that rival Formula One training simulators, where drivers spend 80% of their training time in virtual environments. The same approach could revolutionize surgical education, with AI creating increasingly realistic scenarios that challenge trainees without risking patient safety."

Bernard Marr, "Robots and AI Are Rewriting the Future of Surgery," *Forbes*, September 24, 2025. www.forbes.com.

Strong says the goggles can also help educate patients before surgery. He cites a case in which a patient needed surgery to fix a fracture around his right eye. The surgical team showed the patient 2-D X-ray images and explained how they planned to fix the fracture. But the patient better understood the procedure after seeing a 3-D visual of the surgery in the goggles. According to Strong, "Physicians spend years learning how to piece together many 2D images and then visualize them three-dimensionally. It is impossible to ask patients to do the same thing in 30 minutes. By using this technology, we can give our patients a clear view of what will happen during their surgery."[28]

In addition to bringing hidden objects into view, AI-enhanced vision systems can eliminate blind spots in the operating area. Doctors use lasers, ultrasonic tools, and other electronic devices to destroy tumor tissue and cauterize wounds. The intense heat used in this process burns tissue and creates surgical smoke that obscures a surgeon's view. Algorithms can be trained to perform

A Robot Dentist Called Yomi

Dental extraction surgery is one of the most common medical procedures in the United States. Every year an estimated 20 million Americans have at least one tooth pulled. People who lose a tooth often choose to have a dental implant, which is an artificial tooth that is surgically attached to the jawbone. Most people rely on dental surgeons called periodontists to install implants, but an AI-powered robot named Yomi is taking over the task.

Yomi's AI-powered software reads a patient's CT scan to create an extremely detailed 3-D map of the mouth, skull, and jawbone. The images help the robot pick the exact location, depth, and angle of the implant. Because patients cannot help but move their heads and mouths, Yomi's software reads the smallest movements to aim the drill with high precision. During the procedure, the robot provides feedback to the periodontist, who can intervene if necessary. In 2025 University of Buffalo periodontics professor Nathalia Andrade pointed out that Yomi robots had already been used in more than seventy thousand implant procedures in the United States: "This isn't the future—it's the present. . . . The robot will not . . . make a mistake, such as going too far inside the bone and damaging a critical nerve."

Quoted in Laurie Kaiser, "Robot Demonstrates Dental Implant Procedures," UBNow, University of Buffalo, March 11, 2025. https://dental.buffalo.edu.

dehazing operations that digitally erase smoke from the operating field and provide surgeons with smokeless images in real time.

Autonomous Surgeons

Videos are recorded during operations to allow doctors and researchers to study procedures after completion. Recordings track the exact movements of a surgeon's hands. AI algorithms can be programmed to analyze this data and combine it with motion-tracking datasets created from thousands of other surgeries. This vast amount of data is being used to train robotic surgical equipment that can perform operations autonomously (without human intervention).

In 2025 researchers at Johns Hopkins University created a system called the Hierarchical Surgical Robot Transformer (SRT-H). The AI-powered robot performed autonomous gallbladder removal surgery on a realistic medical dummy with human physiology. Around seven hundred thousand gallbladder removal operations are performed in the United States every year. Doctors performing the procedures are assisted by da Vinci surgery systems.

The Johns Hopkins team was led by robotics researcher Ji Woong Kim and medical roboticist Axel Krieger. The team broke gallbladder surgery down to seventeen specific steps. Using a program similar to ChatGPT, researchers trained the SRT-H system with seventeen hours of gallbladder surgery videos captured by da Vinci cameras. The video feeds were enhanced with kinematics data—the exact motions made by da Vinci's robotic arms. Humans could guide the robotic system with vocal feedback, such as "move your arm a bit to the left."[29]

After training with these vast datasets, the SRT-H system performed operations with a 100 percent success rate. The operations did take longer than those performed by a human surgeon, but

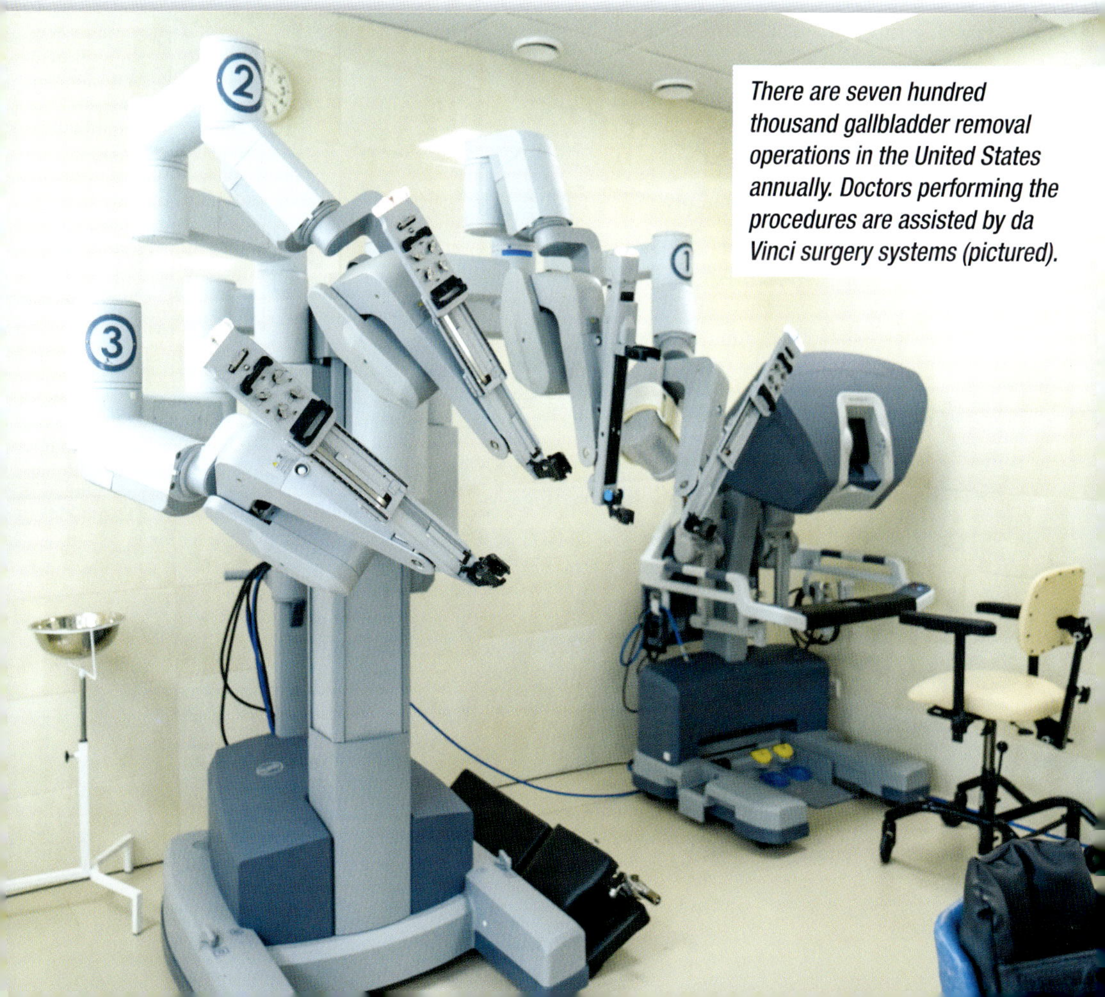

There are seven hundred thousand gallbladder removal operations in the United States annually. Doctors performing the procedures are assisted by da Vinci surgery systems (pictured).

> "The [SRT-H algorithm] told the robot exactly how to move and what to do. It worked like . . . robotic arms welding cars on factory floors."[30]
>
> —Ji Woong Kim, robotics researcher

the results showed promise. And researchers were working to expand the system's capabilities to perform other types of surgery. According to Kim, "The program told the robot exactly how to move and what to do. It worked like . . . robotic arms welding cars on factory floors. . . . You can take any kind of surgery, not just this one, train the robot in the same way, and it will be able to perform that surgery."[30]

Barriers to AI Robotic Surgery

Researchers see great potential for AI-powered surgical robots. Once the machines are perfected, they will be used to perform minor operations, such as hernia repair and even dental surgery. This is expected to lower health care costs, increase success rates, and provide surgeons with more time to perform complex operations. In the future, surgical robots are expected to aid doctors with life-threatening procedures that are now seen as too risky.

The science behind AI-enhanced surgery improves every year. But there are practical problems that need to be solved, especially when it comes to public acceptance. A 2023 poll by the Pew Research Center showed that a majority of Americans were not comfortable turning their health care over to AI algorithms and robots. Nearly 60 percent said they would not want an AI-based surgical robot for their own surgery. The hesitancy can be traced to a general lack of trust in the decision-making capabilities of AI. There are also concerns about the lack of transparency in complex systems that even AI program designers say they sometimes do not fully understand.

People may have doubts about AI in surgery, but big tech companies are moving quickly to incorporate AI into nearly every facet of modern society, including hospital operating rooms. If AI can bring costs down, eliminate human error, and make surgical options available to more people, the general public will doubtlessly learn to accept robots in the operating room.

CHAPTER FIVE

Discovering and Developing New Medicines with AI

Breathing is such a natural process that few people give it much thought. But for the 5 million suffering from a disease called idiopathic pulmonary fibrosis (IPF), every breath is a challenge. IPF is an irreversible disease that causes scarring (fibrosis) in the lungs, which are part of the pulmonary system. The term *idiopathic* indicates that the cause of the condition is unknown. However, those who suffer from IPF experience shortness of breath, chest pain, fatigue, and a persistent dry cough. The condition leads to a loss of independence and restricts simple activities like walking or climbing stairs. IPF can bring about anxiety and depression.

There are drugs that treat some IPF symptoms, but patients who contract the disease can only expect to survive around three years. Drug researchers using AI are working to change the poor prognosis. In 2019 the start-up biotech company Insilico Medicine used AI to design a drug referred to as an antifibrotic small molecule inhibitor. The name indicates that the drug slows down the pace of tissue scarring by targeting a protein molecule responsible for fibrosis. The company created the novel drug and successfully tested it in mice. The prevalidation process took only forty-six days. It now has to conduct clinical trials on humans.

Proteins, Molecules, and Disease

Insilico's accomplishment is notable because creating a new medicinal drug is an extremely complicated and time-consuming process. Researchers most often begin their work by focusing on proteins. These molecules, created from strings of amino acids, perform many functions that are central to building and maintaining life. Proteins transport nutrients, generate and repair tissue, regulate hormones, and are the basis for the antibodies that make up the immune system. Malfunctioning proteins are called misfolded proteins because of the way they are coiled, folded, or tangled like headphone wires in a pocket. Misfolded proteins contain errors in the sequence of amino acids. They are responsible for many diseases, including Parkinson's, a disease of the central nervous system that causes tremors, and Alzheimer's, which results in a decline in memory, personality, and mood. For decades, scientist seeking to cure such diseases used X-ray beams or specialized microscopes to isolate misfolded proteins hidden among millions of other cells. When a misfolded protein could be found, researchers examined it for areas where a drug molecule could bind with it. This process, called molecular binding, cures disease by increasing, decreasing, or blocking a misfolded protein's function. When searching for molecular binding drugs, scientists scrutinize a huge

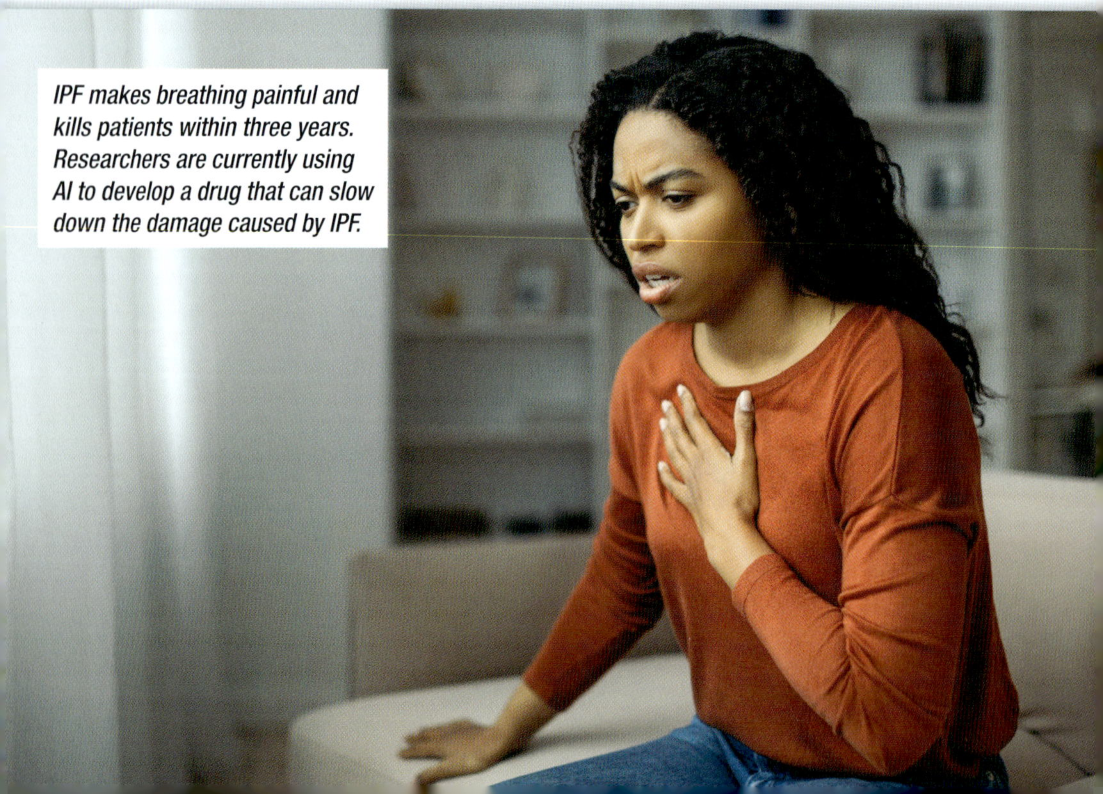

IPF makes breathing painful and kills patients within three years. Researchers are currently using AI to develop a drug that can slow down the damage caused by IPF.

number of compounds. Theories are tested and potential drug molecules are screened for effectiveness.

It can take years of experimental research to find a small number of compounds that show promise as treatments. The compounds are handed over to biologists who test the potential drugs on lab mice. Around 90 percent of the molecules do not work as expected. Insilico was able to disrupt the lengthy, costly molecular binding process with AI. The company employed generative adversarial networks (GANs) to create a new molecule. GANs rely on two AI systems that work against one another to make something new. One network, called the generator, processed databases of around thirty thousand possible drug molecules at speeds far beyond human capabilities. Substances that might be useful for further research were identified. A second network, called the discriminator, focused on what is called predictive analysis. Its algorithms predicted which generated drug candidates might be effective and how they might behave in complex biological systems.

> **"We are eager to continue to advance this potentially first-in-class [IPF] therapy forward to help patients in need and show the value of generative AI in drug discovery and development."[31]**
>
> —Alex Zhavoronkov, founder of Insilico Medicine

The GANs created chemical structures for six molecules that might target the folded protein that causes lung scarring in IPF patients. Of this number, a drug called INS018_055 was found to alter the protein and slow the disease. In 2023 company founder Alex Zhavoronkov issued a statement about the new drug: "When we started developing generative AI for drug discovery, I never expected to see the . . . results we have today. . . . We are eager to continue to advance this potentially first-in-class therapy forward to help patients in need and show the value of generative AI in drug discovery and development."[31]

Healing on a Cellular Level

Generative AI follows the traditional drug discovery route, seeking to change single proteins that cause illness. But some diseases

Cracking the Protein Puzzle

Proteins are molecules made up of long chains of amino acids, and they are central to all life on Earth. There are hundreds of millions of various proteins found in people, plants, animals, and even bacteria. A protein's function is linked to its shape, but scientists using traditional methods have been unable to map very many 3-D protein structures. This has long been a problem for medical researchers. Errors within proteins create misfolded proteins, which are responsible for numerous diseases. Scientists seeking to cure diseases need to understand a protein's 3-D structure to devise drugs that can change a protein's shape or destroy it.

An AI program called AlphaFold, released by Google DeepMind in 2022, is seen as a drug research game changer. The program was used to create an open-source database that predicted the 3-D structures of over 200 million proteins. Researchers using AlphaFold gained new insights into Parkinson's disease and were able to create an improved malaria vaccine. According to Demis Hassabis, founder and chief executive officer of DeepMind, "AlphaFold is the singular and momentous advance in life science that demonstrates the power of AI. Determining the 3-D structure of a protein used to take many months or years, it now takes seconds."

Demis Hassabis, "AlphaFold Reveals the Structure of the Protein Universe," Google DeepMind, July 28, 2022. https://deepmind.google.

are triggered by genetic mutations, which are malfunctions in the genes that are contained in cells. Malfunctioning cells can interact with proteins and healthy cells and cause diseases in ways that scientists do not fully understand. Researchers at Harvard University wanted to learn more about these interactions to develop new therapies and drug treatments. This led them to develop an AI tool called a PDGrapher.

The PDGrapher can analyze specific genes and cells to learn whether they are healthy or diseased. The system creates AI models that show researchers what would happen if some of the cellular parts were turned off or modified in some way. With this information, the PDGrapher can pinpoint which genes to target with drugs in order to return the cells to a healthy state. The senior researcher on the Harvard project, Marinka Zitnik, a professor of biomedical informatics, uses a cooking metaphor to explain the PDGrapher:

Traditional drug discovery resembles tasting hundreds of prepared dishes to find one that happens to taste perfect. . . . PDGrapher works like a master chef who understands what they want the dish to be and exactly how to combine ingredients to achieve the desired flavor. . . . Instead of testing every possible recipe, PDGrapher asks: "Which mix of ingredients will turn this bland or overly salty dish into a perfectly balanced meal?"[32]

Researchers say the accuracy of the PDGrapher is superior to other AI tools used in drug research. It has been found to be particularly useful for studying Parkinson's and Alzheimer's, which are complex diseases fueled by multiple biological factors. Scientists predict that one day the PDGrapher will be used to develop cellular profiles of individual patients. This will allow doctors to design novel treatment combinations for each person. Zitnik says, "Our ultimate goal is to create a clear road map of possible ways to reverse disease at the cellular level."[33]

> **"Traditional drug discovery resembles tasting hundreds of prepared dishes to find one that happens to taste perfect. . . . [The AI tool] PDGrapher works like a master chef who understands what they want the dish to be and exactly how to combine ingredients to achieve the desired flavor."[32]**
>
> —Marinka Zitnik, professor of biomedical informatics

Seeking Cancer Cures

In 2025 a different sort of AI cell profile program was being developed at Yale University. Researchers are hoping to use the tool, called the Archetypal Analysis network (AAnet), to better understand the types of cells found in tumors that cause breast, lung, and other types of cancer. Common cancer treatments include chemotherapy (drugs that shrink or kill cancer cells) and radiation therapy (using high-energy rays to eliminate cancerous cells). Both types of treatment have unpleasant side effects, including chronic fatigue, hair loss, and severe nausea.

The problem is that cancer tumors are composed of different types of cells. One type of therapy might kill most cells but not all

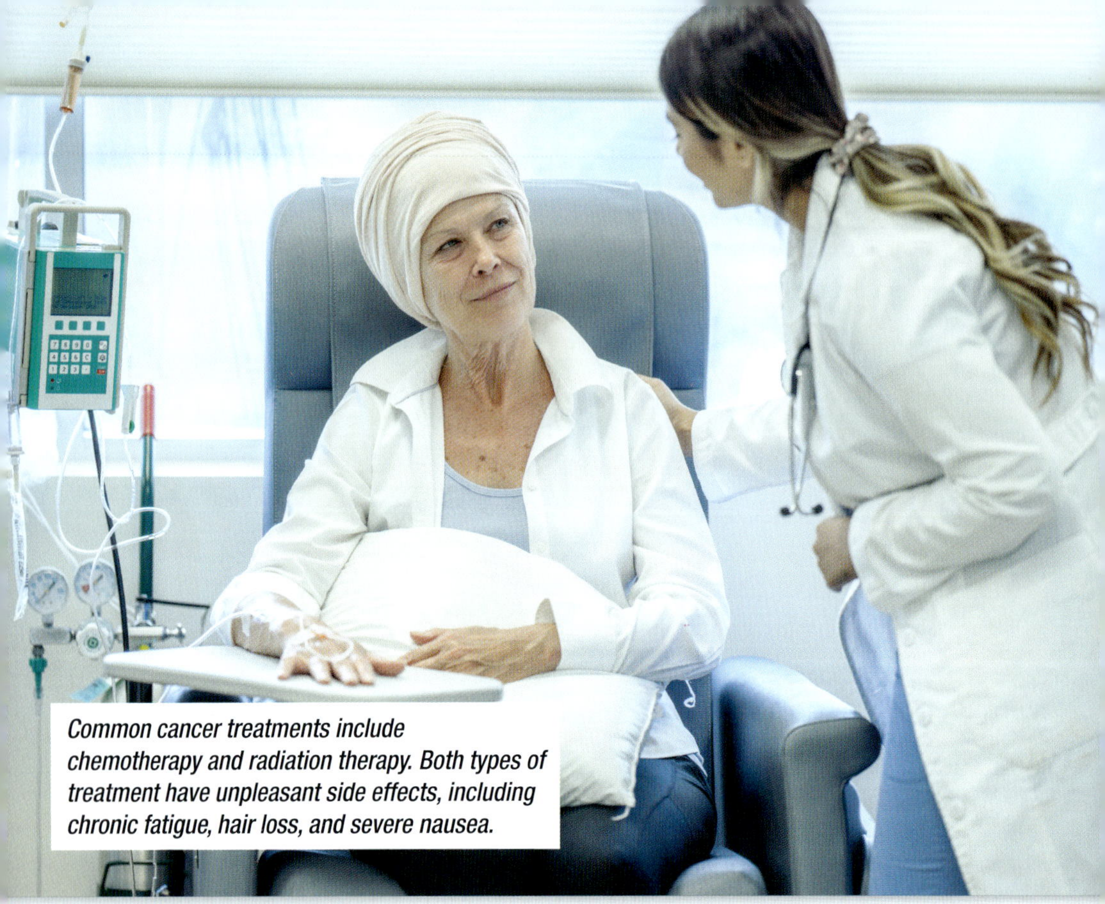

Common cancer treatments include chemotherapy and radiation therapy. Both types of treatment have unpleasant side effects, including chronic fatigue, hair loss, and severe nausea.

of them. And the remaining cells can continue to grow, allowing the cancer to return. According to cancer researcher Christine L. Chaffer, "So far researchers haven't been able to clearly explain how adjacent cells in a tumor differ from each other, and how to classify those differences into meaningful ways to better treat tumors. But this is exactly what we need to know so we can kill all cells within that tumor with the right therapies."[34]

> "So far researchers haven't been able to clearly explain how adjacent cells in a tumor differ from each other, and how to classify those differences into meaningful ways to better treat tumors. But this is exactly what we need to know so we can kill all cells within that tumor with the right therapies."[34]
>
> —Christine L. Chaffer, cancer researcher

AAnet is helping researchers identify the diverse cells found in tumors. The program has been used to detect patterns in the genes of individual cells of breast cancer tumors. AAnet identified five unique cancer cell groups within a single tumor. According to Chaffer,

> Each group exhibited different biological pathways and propensities for growth. . . . Our next steps are to see how these groups may change over time, for example before and after chemotherapy. . . . With AAnet, we now hope to . . . design combination therapies that we know will target each of those different groups through their biological pathways. This has the potential to vastly improve outcomes for that patient.[35]

A Slow, Tedious Process

Tools like AAnet and PDGrapher can help researchers develop new drug treatments. But even when a miraculous new medicine is discovered, it can take years before it is available to patients. This is due to grindingly slow processes required to bring new drugs to market. Doctors hope that AI can be used to make this process faster and more efficient.

In the United States, the FDA sets quality standards for many products, including pharmaceutical drugs. The FDA requires any new prescription medicine to undergo a rigorous three-part procedure called a clinic drug trial. During phase one, the medication is given to healthy volunteers. If they do not experience harmful side effects, the drug trial enters phase two, when it is given to people who suffer from the condition the drug is meant to treat. If these volunteers get better, or do not get sicker, the drug trial enters phase three. In this final phase, the drug is provided to a large and diverse group of people suffering from the illness. According to science writer Vanessa Bates Ramirez, "Out of more than a million screened molecules, on average just one makes it to late stage clinical trials and ends up getting approved for use."[36]

In 2025 Insilico's vice president of clinical development, Carol Satler, was still overseeing phase two of the clinical trial for the IPF drug. She was working with a team of highly paid doctors, clinical researchers, data managers, lab workers, statisticians, and others needed to manage the complex FDA requirements. And the process required Satler to continually seek out new patients, one by one over months and years, who would best benefit from a phase three trial. As Satler said, "The meter is always running. It's so expensive."[37]

Virtual Patients

AI researchers are taking aim at drug development barriers in two ways. The first is meant to benefit drug trial volunteers who are often required to make frequent visits to clinics over an extended time period. This inconvenience results in test subjects dropping out of trials, which can skew the final results. AI can reduce this problem through the use of remote monitoring. AI-powered apps and wearable devices allow doctors to collect data while trial participants are at home or at work. In addition to retaining volunteers, remote monitoring increases accuracy—visits to a clinic can increase stress levels and raise a patient's blood pressure, which can impact the trial results.

AI Drug Manufacturing

In 2025 the Utah-based pharmaceutical company Recursion was using AI to create a new drug that promises to slow the growth of blood cancer cells. The process requires scientists to create test drugs from individual atoms. This is done in an AI-powered robotic drug production facility, which science journalist Veronique Greenwood describes:

> One cold morning late last year, I went to see one of Recursion's discovery engines. . . . [It is in] a room the size of a small supermarket with aisles of machines in plate-glass cases. White lamps like halos hung above them. "We've got biology on one side, chemistry on the other," [Patrick Collins, the director of automation] said. A magnetic railway threaded through the machines, connecting . . . robots to incubator chambers. . . . [These machines] dispense molecules created from raw atoms, molecules that AI systems have already tested and explored in virtual spaces. The candidate drugs drip onto trays of cells, and the system evaluates their effects. It's new, and there are kinks to be worked out. Some parts of the automated process still need humans to move them along. . . . But when it works, scientists will have the results of thousands of tests glowing on their screens . . . helping to make future drugs.

Veronique Greenwood, "Where Are All the AI Drugs?," *Wired*, July 17, 2025. www.wired.com.

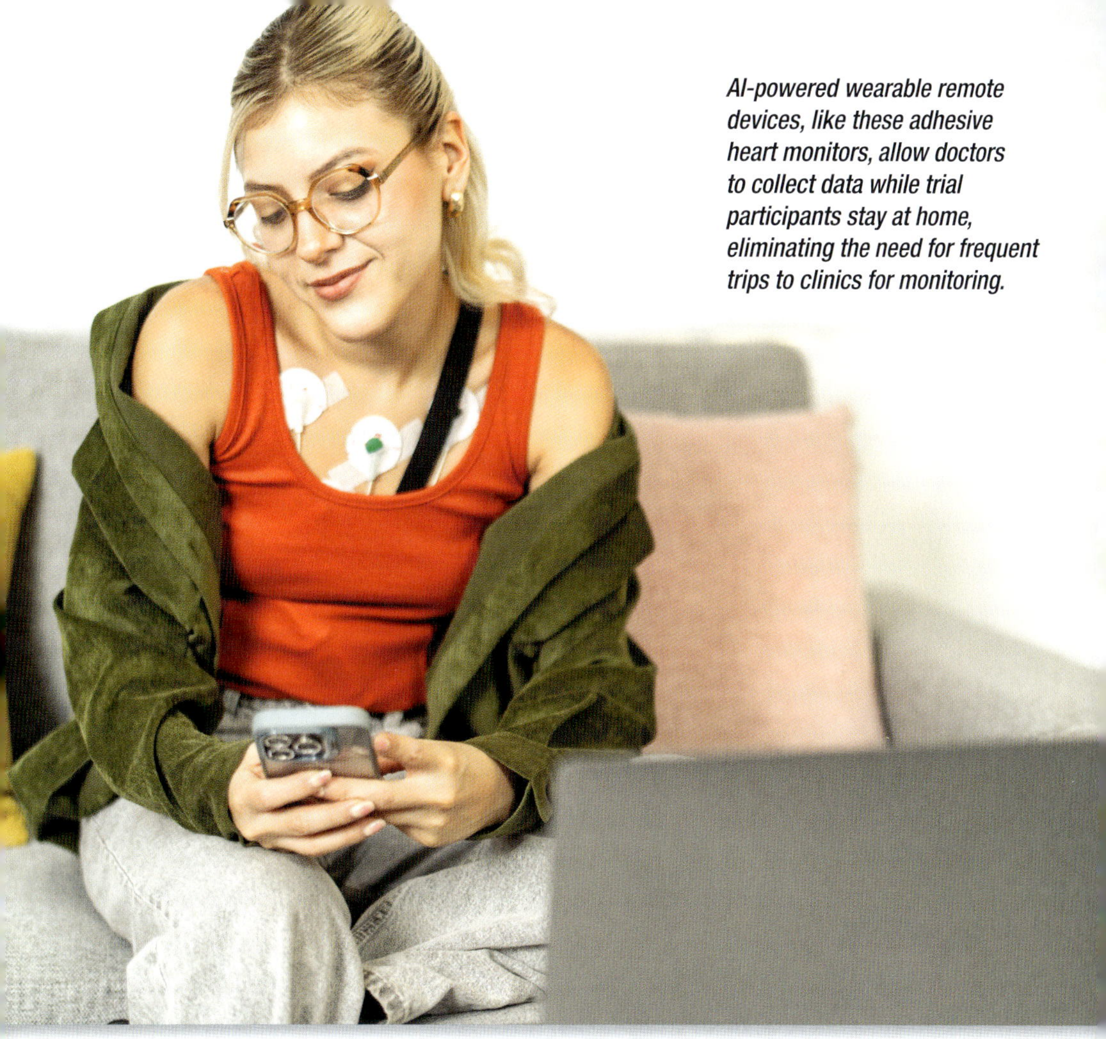

AI-powered wearable remote devices, like these adhesive heart monitors, allow doctors to collect data while trial participants stay at home, eliminating the need for frequent trips to clinics for monitoring.

Remote monitoring is beneficial for use in conventional clinical trials. But researchers in France are using AI to make the entire drug trial process shorter and cheaper. They are eliminating humans from the equation altogether and testing new drugs on virtual patients. This process, known as agent-based modeling, creates computer-generated test subjects that imitate the characteristics of real patients. These models can be used to simulate therapeutic drug trials, test rare drug interactions, and model drug treatments that can be used in a wide range of different real-world physical conditions.

Researchers creating a virtual patient use clinical data from people with the disease. The GANs create virtual patients by scanning reams of historic medical data, including disease symptoms, weight, medication history, and genetic information. This literature helps AI programs create charts, graphs, and other information for use by scientists. The virtual patients can be divided into groups by gender, lineage, and other features. Each virtual group can be tested with new drugs to determine side effects, dosage levels, and effectiveness.

In 2023 agent-based modeling was used in cancer research to simulate tumors in virtual patients. The AI program was able to track the progression of tumor growth and judge the effects of different therapies used alone and together. This enabled researchers to predict the value of medicines used in a variety of scenarios.

Challenges Remain

AI is rapidly transforming drug research and development from start-ups such as Insilico to respected universities and major drug companies. Scientists harnessing the power of AI are identifying and testing effective drugs more rapidly and finding more efficient ways to treat destructive diseases that have haunted humanity for centuries.

SOURCE NOTES

Introduction: Transformative Technology

1. Quoted in Dani Blum and Maggie Astor, "White House Health Report Included Fake Citations," *New York Times,* May 29, 2025. www.nytimes.com.
2. Quoted in Blum and Astor, "White House Health Report Included Fake Citations."
3. Quoted in Baptist Health, "The Promises and Pitfalls of AI in Medicine," March 25, 2025. https://physicianresources.baptisthealth.net.
4. Leana S. Wen, "'Stethoscopes in the Sand': Why I'm Rethinking AI's Role in Medicine," *Washington Post,* October 7, 2025. www.washingtonpost.com.
5. Quoted in Steven Lohr, "Your A.I. Radiologist Will Not Be with You Soon," *New York Times,* May 14, 2025. www.nytimes.com.

Chapter One: AI in Mental Health

6. Quoted in Nicole Levine, "An AI Ally for Mental Health," *Cedars-Sinai Magazine,* April 16, 2024. www.cedars-sinai.org.
7. Quoted in Emily Woodruff, "Doctors at Cedars-Sinai Develop AI-Powered Mental Health 'Robot' Therapist," *Los Angeles Times,* July 22, 2025. www.latimes.com.
8. Quoted in Gaby Clark, ed., "AI Technology for Early Screening of Autism Spectrum Disorder Developed," Medical Xpress, June 23, 2025. https://medicalxpress.com.
9. Quoted in Sarah Wells, "An AI Social Coach Is Teaching Empathy to People with Autism," Stanford Human-Centered Artificial Intelligence, August 13, 2025. https://hai.stanford.edu.
10. Quoted in Wells, "An AI Social Coach Is Teaching Empathy to People with Autism."
11. Quoted in Tyler Francischine, "AI-Powered Clinical Tool Aims to Prevent Opioid Disorder Relapse," University of Florida College of Pharmacy, October 9, 2025. https://pharmacy.ufl.edu.
12. Quoted in Harini Barath, "AI Tools Reveal Knowledge Gaps in Addiction Treatment," Dartmouth College, February 22, 2024. https://home.dartmouth.edu.

13. Quoted in Sarah Wells, "Exploring the Dangers of AI in Mental Health Care," Stanford Human-Centered Artificial Intelligence, June 11, 2025. https://hai.stanford.edu.

Chapter Two: A New Era in Detecting Disease

14. Charlotte Blease, *Dr. Bot.* Yale University Press, 2025, p. 12.
15. Quoted in Julie Galante, "Using AI to Combat Medical Misdiagnosis and Improve Patient Care," Harvard Kennedy School, March 18, 2024. www.hks.harvard.edu.
16. Quoted in Galante, "Using AI to Combat Medical Misdiagnosis and Improve Patient Care."
17. Quoted in Alvin Powell, "Machine Healing," *Harvard Gazette,* March 30, 2025. https://news.harvard.edu.
18. Adam Rodman, "Can AI Make Medicine More Human?," *Harvard Medicine Magazine,* Autumn 2024. https://magazine.hms.harvard .edu.

Chapter Three: AI and Personalized Medicine

19. Quoted in Kate Morgan, "Doctors Told Him He Was Going to Die. Then A.I. Saved His Life," *New York Times,* March 20, 2025. www .nytimes.com.
20. Quoted in Morgan, "Doctors Told Him He Was Going to Die."
21. Quoted in Rebecca Handler, "MedStory: Revolutionizing Cancer Diagnosis with SEQUOIA," Stanford Medicine, February 15, 2025. https://med.stanford.edu.
22. Quoted in Alana Wyche, "Cleveland Clinic–Led Research Shows How AI-Supported Precision Health and Lifestyle Coaching Program Can Improve Outcomes in Patients with Type 2 Diabetes," Cleveland Clinic Newsroom, August 20, 2025. https://newsroom .clevelandclinic.org.

Chapter Four: Transforming Surgery with AI

23. Quoted in Chris Gayomali, "Meet Sturgeon, the AI Tool That Helps Doctors Identify Brain Tumors Faster than Ever," *National Geographic,* October 15, 2024. www.nationalgeographic.com.
24. Quoted in Noah Fromson, "In 10 Seconds, AI Model Detects Cancerous Brain Tumor Often Missed During Surgery," Michigan Medicine, November 13, 2024. www.michiganmedicine.org.
25. Bernard Marr, "Robots and AI Are Rewriting the Future of Surgery," *Forbes,* September 24, 2025. www.forbes.com.

26. Quoted in Marr, "Robots and AI Are Rewriting the Future of Surgery."
27. Quoted in Liam Connolly, "The Future of Surgery: Using Augmented Reality Goggles in the Operating Room," UC Davis Health, August 8, 2024. https://health.ucdavis.edu.
28. Quoted in Connolly, "The Future of Surgery."
29. Quoted in Jacek Krywko, "Experimental Surgery Performed by AI-Driven Surgical Robot," Ars Technica, July 21, 2025. https://arstechnica.com.
30. Quoted in Krywko, "Experimental Surgery Performed by AI-Driven Surgical Robot."

Chapter Five: Discovering and Developing New Medicines with AI

31. Quoted in Brita Bell, "First Drug Discovered and Designed with Generative AI Enters Phase II Trials, with First Patients Dosed," EurekAlert!, American Association for the Advancement of Science, June 27, 2023. www.eurekalert.org.
32. Quoted in Ekaterina Pesheva, "New AI Tool Pinpoints Genes, Drug Combo to Restore Health in Diseased Cells," Harvard Medical School, September 9, 2025. https://hms.harvard.edu.
33. Quoted in Pesheva, "New AI Tool Pinpoints Genes, Drug Combo to Restore Health in Diseased Cells."
34. Quoted in Yale Engineering, "AI Tool Set to Transform Characterization and Treatment of Cancers," June 24, 2025. https://engineering.yale.edu.
35. Quoted in Yale Engineering, "AI Tool Set to Transform Characterization and Treatment of Cancers."
36. Vanessa Bates Ramirez, "In a First, an AI-Designed Drug Is Being Tested in Humans to See If It Actually Works," Singularity Hub, June 28, 2023. https://singularityhub.com.
37. Quoted in Veronique Greenwood, "Where Are All the AI Drugs?," *Wired,* July 17, 2025. www.wired.com.

FOR FURTHER RESEARCH

Books

John Allen, *Artificial Intelligence: Promise and Peril*. ReferencePoint, 2024.

Martha Brockenbrough, *Future Tense: How We Made Artificial Intelligence—and How It Will Change Everything*. Feiwel & Friends, 2024.

Matt Greenwood, *Artificial Intelligence: An Introduction to AI for Teenagers.* Ochreland, 2024.

Lynn Raebsamen, *Artificial Stupelligence: The Hilarious Truth About AI*. Lyra, 2025.

Shah Rukh, *Artificial Intelligence in Healthcare*. Published by the author, 2023.

Internet Resources

Chris Gayomali, "Meet Sturgeon, the AI Tool That Helps Doctors Identify Brain Tumors Faster than Ever," *National Geographic*, October 15, 2024. www.nationalgeographic.com.

Veronique Greenwood, "Where Are All the AI Drugs?," *Wired*, July 17, 2025. www.wired.com.

Kate Morgan, "Doctors Told Him He Was Going to Die. Then A.I. Saved His Life," *New York Times*, March 20, 2025. www.nytimes.com.

Sarah Wells, "An AI Social Coach Is Teaching Empathy to People with Autism," Stanford Human-Centered Artificial Intelligence, August 13, 2025. https://hai.stanford.edu.

Leana S. Wen, "'Stethoscopes in the Sand': Why I'm Rethinking AI's Role in Medicine," *Washington Post*, October 7, 2025. www.washingtonpost.com.

Websites

Harvard Gazette

https://news.harvard.edu

The "Health" and "Science & Tech" sections of the *Harvard Gazette* cover the latest university research into gene mapping, AI, and other pertinent issues.

Journal of Medical Artificial Intelligence (JMAI)
https://jmai.amegroups.org
The *JMAI* focuses on the use of AI in nearly every aspect of the medical field. The scholarly, open-access articles provide insights into AI research, robotic surgery, and data analytics and mining.

MedLinePlus Magazine
https://magazine.medlineplus.gov
This online health information resource, hosted by the National Institutes of Health, features information about AI, various diseases, genetics, pharmaceutical drugs, and medical testing.

Medscape
www.medscape.com
Medscape offers articles and videos that cover the latest medical news, drug and disease updates, and emerging uses of AI in health care.

Science
www.science.org/journal/science
This site, hosted by the American Association for the Advancement of Science, covers recent scientific discoveries, including the latest news about AI, medicine, and robotics. The site features blogs, commentary, and analysis.

INDEX

Note: Boldface page numbers indicate illustrations.